THE RANDOMIZED CLINICAL TRIAL
AND THERAPEUTIC DECISIONS

STATISTICS: Textbooks and Monographs

A SERIES EDITED BY

D. B. OWEN, Coordinating Editor
*Department of Statistics
Southern Methodist University
Dallas, Texas*

R. G. CORNELL, Associate Editor for Biostatistics
*School of Public Health
University of Michigan
Ann Arbor, Michigan*

Vol. 1: The Generalized Jackknife Statistic, *H. L. Gray and W. R. Schucany*
Vol. 2: Multivariate Analysis, *Anant M. Kshirsagar*
Vol. 3: Statistics and Society, *Walter T. Federer*
Vol. 4: Multivariate Analysis: A Selected and Abstracted Bibliography, 1957-1972, *Kocherlakota Subrahmaniam and Kathleen Subrahmaniam* (out of print)
Vol. 5: Design of Experiments: A Realistic Approach, *Virgil L. Anderson and Robert A. McLean*
Vol. 6: Statistical and Mathematical Aspects of Pollution Problems, *John W. Pratt*
Vol. 7: Introduction to Probability and Statistics (in two parts), Part I: Probability; Part II: Statistics, *Narayan C. Giri*
Vol. 8: Statistical Theory of the Analysis of Experimental Designs, *J. Ogawa*
Vol. 9: Statistical Techniques in Simulation (in two parts), *Jack P. C. Kleijnen*
Vol. 10: Data Quality Control and Editing, *Joseph I. Naus*
Vol. 11: Cost of Living Index Numbers: Practice, Precision, and Theory, *Kali S. Banerjee*
Vol. 12: Weighing Designs: For Chemistry, Medicine, Economics, Operations Research, Statistics, *Kali S. Banerjee*
Vol. 13: The Search for Oil: Some Statistical Methods and Techniques, *edited by D. B. Owen*
Vol. 14: Sample Size Choice: Charts for Experiments with Linear Models, *Robert E. Odeh and Martin Fox*
Vol. 15: Statistical Methods for Engineers and Scientists, *Robert M. Bethea, Benjamin S. Duran, and Thomas L. Boullion*
Vol. 16: Statistical Quality Control Methods, *Irving W. Burr*
Vol. 17: On the History of Statistics and Probability, *edited by D. B. Owen*
Vol. 18: Econometrics, *Peter Schmidt*
Vol. 19: Sufficient Statistics: Selected Contributions, *Vasant S. Huzurbazar (edited by Anant M. Kshirsagar)*
Vol. 20: Handbook of Statistical Distributions, *Jagdish K. Patel, C. H. Kapadia, and D. B. Owen*
Vol. 21: Case Studies in Sample Design, *A. C. Rosander*

Vol. 22: Pocket Book of Statistical Tables, *compiled by R. E. Odeh, D. B. Owen, Z. W. Birnbaum, and L. Fisher*
Vol. 23: The Information in Contingency Tables, *D. V. Gokhale and Solomon Kullback*
Vol. 24: Statistical Analysis of Reliability and Life-Testing Models: Theory and Methods, *Lee J. Bain*
Vol. 25: Elementary Statistical Quality Control, *Irving W. Burr*
Vol. 26: An Introduction to Probability and Statistics Using BASIC, *Richard A. Groeneveld*
Vol. 27: Basic Applied Statistics, *B. L. Raktoe and J. J. Hubert*
Vol. 28: A Primer in Probability, *Kathleen Subrahmaniam*
Vol. 29: Random Processes: A First Look, *R. Syski*
Vol. 30: Regression Methods: A Tool for Data Analysis, *Rudolf J. Freund and Paul D. Minton*
Vol. 31: Randomization Tests, *Eugene S. Edgington*
Vol. 32: Tables for Normal Tolerance Limits, Sampling Plans, and Screening, *Robert E. Odeh and D. B. Owen*
Vol. 33: Statistical Computing, *William J. Kennedy, Jr. and James E. Gentle*
Vol. 34: Regression Analysis and Its Application: A Data-Oriented Approach, *Richard F. Gunst and Robert L. Mason*
Vol. 35: Scientific Strategies to Save Your Life, *I. D. J. Bross*
Vol. 36: Statistics in the Pharmaceutical Industry, *edited by C. Ralph Buncher and Jia-Yeong Tsay*
Vol. 37: Sampling from a Finite Population, *J. Hájek*
Vol. 38: Statistical Modeling Techniques, *S. S. Shapiro*
Vol. 39: Statistical Theory and Inference in Research, *T. A. Bancroft and C.-P. Han*
Vol. 40: Handbook of the Normal Distribution, *Jagdish K. Patel and Campbell B. Read*
Vol. 41: Recent Advances in Regression Methods, *Hrishikesh D. Vinod and Aman Ullah*
Vol. 42: Acceptance Sampling in Quality Control, *Edward G. Schilling*
Vol. 43: The Randomized Clinical Trial and Therapeutic Decisions, *edited by Niels Tygstrup, John M. Lachin, and Erik Juhl*

OTHER VOLUMES IN PREPARATION

THE RANDOMIZED CLINICAL TRIAL AND THERAPEUTIC DECISIONS

Edited by
NIELS TYGSTRUP
Rigshospitalet
University of Copenhagen
Copenhagen, Denmark

JOHN M. LACHIN
The Biostatistics Center
Department of Statistics
The George Washington University
Washington, D.C.

ERIK JUHL
Hvidovre Hospital
University of Copenhagen
Copenhagen, Denmark

MARCEL DEKKER, INC.   New York and Basel

Library of Congress Cataloging in Publication Data
Main entry under title:

The Randomized clinical trial and therapeutic decisions.

(Statistics, textbooks and monographs; v. 43)
Includes bibliographies and index.
1. Therapeutics--Decision-making. 2. Therapeutics, Experimental
--Statistical methods.   3. Medicine, Clinical--Research--Statistical
methods. 4. Statistical decisions. I. Tygstrup, Niels. II. Lachin, John
M., (date). III. Juhl, Erik, (date). IV. Series. (DNLM: 1. Clinical trials.
2. Research design. W20.5 R194)
RM103.R18 1982   615.5'0724   82-8971
ISBN 0-8247-1856-9   AACR2

COPYRIGHT © 1982 by MARCEL DEKKER, INC.
ALL RIGHTS RESERVED

Neither this book nor any part may be reproduced or transmitted in any form or by any means, electronic or mechanical, including photocopying, microfilming, and recording, or by any information storage and retrieval system, without permission in writing from the publisher.

MARCEL DEKKER, INC.
270 Madison Avenue, New York, New York 10016

Current printing (last digit):
10 9 8 7 6 5 4 3 2 1

PRINTED IN THE UNITED STATES OF AMERICA

Dedicated to

Franz J. Ingelfinger

in Memoriam

Foreword

The idea for this book was born in Varenna, a little town on the lake of Como, Northern Italy. The Italian Society of Gastroenterology had planned an educational intervention on research applied to medical care. Too few clinical studies were being conducted in the gastroenterological milieu of Italy. We needed first to form more investigators who knew how the rationale for bedside therapeutic or diagnostic decisions could be properly addressed in a scientific protocol.

The course in Varenna, planned and directed by Niels Tygstrup, was a masterpiece of work in scientific formation. From the first day, all participants realized how far the course was removed from routine postgraduate courses, meetings, or congresses. The quiet atmosphere of the ancient Villa Monastero, where Fermi once taught physics, and the continuous interaction and balance among the members of the faculty and between the faculty and the students created a kind of magic harmony of design and proportions, of information and critical skill. Such events are unfortunately rare in rituals used among physicians and investigators.

The text of the book has been updated thanks to the hard efforts of the editors and faculty, but all the flavor of the course has been preserved.

The Society thanks the thirty students, who demonstrated how eager young investigators are to adopt a scientific approach for new problems in medical care. Thanks also to Franco B. Bianchi, Paolo A. Bianchi, Lucio Capurso, Livio Chiandussi, Maurizio M. Koch, Ivano Lorenzini, Federico Manenti, and Luigi Pagliaro, who contributed to the course by acting as tutors of the students, and to the Ente Villa Monastero, Como, Italy.

FRANCESCO ORLANDI
Department of Gastroenterology
School of Medicine and General Hospital
Ancona, Italy

Preface

In the recent past randomized clinical trials have had increasing impact on clinical practice and therapeutic decisions. Previously, however, therapeutic decisions were often made without guidance from randomized clinical trials, simply because relevant trials were lacking. This is changing with the increasing number of trials being conducted. What may be more important, however, is that the randomized clinical trial is being accepted as a tool for the solution of therapeutic problems, which in turn represents an approval of the classical scientific approach to clinical practice. The general success of scientific methodology in the aquisition of new knowledge gives promise that the randomized clinical trial will have a significant impact on medical care.

In principle, the randomized clinical trial resembles the manner in which clinicians have always gained skills and experience, i.e., by systematic, not random, trial and error. The difference lies in the increase in precision offered by the clinical trial. By systematic collection and analysis of relevant data, the clinical trial attempts to quantify therapeutic effects in comparative terms. The risk of reaching a wrong conclusion is not eliminated, but usually it is smaller (and always better defined) than when therapeutic evaluations are based on general impressions, anecdotal experience, or beliefs. Furthermore, the need for precision regarding criteria for selection of patients and evaluation of therapeutic effects in clinical trials serves to reveal where current diagnostic concepts and therapeutic objectives are inaccurate or irreproducible.

On the other hand, the randomized clinical trial brings into focus the dilemma between an individual-orientated clinical practice and a group-orientated scientific approach. This is a problem not just for those who conduct clinical trials, but perhaps much more so for the clinicians who wish to make therapeutic decisions based on the results of clinical trials, i.e., the "consumers" of trials. Without a certain knowledge of the methodology of clinical trials, the background, the limitations, and the pitfalls, the consumers may easily be mislead.

This book is not intended to be a handbook on the conduct of clinical trials. It does not pretend to give the complete recipe of how to conduct a trial, even though we hope that it will encourage more physicians to engage in such activity. The intention is to provide the consumers and prospective participants, perhaps including patients, with an understanding of the mechanism of a clinical trial and the kind of information it yields, so that they can interpret, evaluate, and apply its results critically. It is meant to be armchair reading, even if some parts may need a little desk work to be properly digested.

We felt that this material, originating from a postgraduate course, provides a particularly favorable basis for this approach because of the many diadactic repetitions, viewing the same basic elements of a clinical trial from different angles--at first simple, later more complex. Furthermore, we find it extremely valuable to be able to include the discussions among the faculty members. They remind the reader that there is still room for differences of opinion, and despite highly needed refinements of methodology, many loose ends remain. It also shows, however, that there is little disagreement about the fundamental principles through which clinical practice, biostatistics, and medical ethics are harmoniously unified in a well-conceived and -executed clinical trial. The message is that the randomized clinical trial starts and ends at the bedside.

We are greatly indebted to the Italian Society of Gastroenterology for arranging the course on which this book is based, to the faculty members for their willingness to transform their lectures into manuscripts in accordance with the scope of the book, and to the students who during the course helped us to keep the scope in mind.

The initial course was developed by Dr. Tygstrup and Dr. Juhl who then supervised the transcription of the proceedings and the initial editing of the manuscript. The final manuscript was largely edited and prepared by Dr. Lachin and additional material was then added, including Chapter 11. We wish to thank Mrs. Sonnia Tidwell for the diligent preparation of the final manuscript; and Professors Lawrence Shaw, Nathan Mantel, Max Halperin, and Peter Thall for their comments on prior drafts.

NIELS TYGSTRUP
JOHN M. LACHIN
ERIK JUHL

Contributors

ANDRÉ L. BLUM, M.D. Medical Clinic, Triemli Hospital, Zurich, Switzerland

THOMAS C. CHALMERS, M.D. The Mount Sinai Medical Center, Mount Sinai School of Medicine, New York, New York

FRANZ J. INGELFINGER, M.D.† The New England Journal of Medicine, Boston, Massachusetts

ERIK JUHL, M.D. Medical Department, Division of Hepatology, Hvidovre Hospital, University of Copenhagen, Copenhagen, Denmark

JOHN M. LACHIN, Sc.D. The Biostatistics Center, Department of Statistics, The George Washington University, Washington, D.C.

AVIVA PETRIE, M.Sc.* Department of Medical Statistics and Epidemiology, London School of Hygiene and Tropical Medicine, and Department of Medical Statistics, Royal Postgraduate Medical School, London, England

POVL RIIS, M.D. Department of Internal Medicine, Herlev Hospital, University of Copenhagen, Copenhagen, Denmark

---

†Dr. Ingelfinger is deceased.
*Ms. Petrie is currently with the London School of Hygiene and Tropical Medicine, London, England.

LESLIE J. SCHOENFIELD, M.D. Department of Gastroenterology, Cedars-Sinai Medical Center, University of California at Los Angeles, Los Angeles, California

NIELS TYGSTRUP, M.D. Medical Department, Division of Hepatology, Rigshospitalet, University of Copenhagen, Copenhagen, Denmark

RALPH WRIGHT, M.D. Medical Unit, The University of Southampton, Southampton General Hospital, Southampton, England

Contents

Foreword   Francesco Orlandi   v

Preface   vii

Contributors   xi

Part I: THE RELATION BETWEEN CLINICAL MEDICINE
AND THE RANDOMIZED CLINICAL TRIAL

1. How Therapeutic Decisions Are Motivated   3
    Povl Riis
    1.1   Introduction 3
    1.2   Discussion 6
          References 10
          Additional Readings 11

2. The Randomized Clinical Trial as a Basis
    for Therapeutic Decisions   13
    Thomas C. Chalmers
    2.1   Introduction 13
    2.2   Discussion 15
          References 19
          Additional Readings 19

xiv Contents

3. Contributions of Randomized Clinical Trials over a
   Decade (1964-1973) to Gastroenterological Therapy   21
   Erik Juhl

   3.1 Introduction 21
   3.2 Discussion 29
        References 30
        Additional Reading 30

Part II: CLINICAL FUNDAMENTALS OF THE RANDOMIZED CLINICAL TRIAL

4. Clinical Elements of the Randomized Clinical Trial   33
   Erik Juhl

   4.1 Patient Selection 33
   4.2 Random Allocation 34
   4.3 Treatment Period 35
   4.4 Statistical Analysis 37
   4.5 Discussion 38
        References 41
        Additional Readings 41

5. Principles for Selection and Exclusion   43
   André L. Blum

   5.1 A Laboratory Experiment 43
   5.2 The Clinical Trial 46
   5.3 Prognostic Stratification 49
   5.4 Compliance 52
   5.5 Discussion 52
        References 57

6. Clinical Evaluation of Success   59
   André L. Blum

   6.1 Multiple Factors 59
   6.2 Clinical Impressions 61
   6.3 Direct versus Indirect Measures
        of Therapeutic Effects 62
   6.4 Clinical Scores 63
   6.5 Stratification 65
   6.6 Premature Exits from Study 67
   6.7 Compliance 69
   6.8 Discussion 71
        References 73

Part III: STATISTICAL FUNDAMENTALS OF THE RANDOMIZED CLINICAL TRIAL

7. Statistical Elements of the Randomized Clinical Trial 77

   John M. Lachin

   7.1 The Clinical Trial 77
   7.2 Design 78
   7.3 Sample Size 88
   7.4 Execution 92
   7.5 Ethics 95
   7.6 Analysis 95
   7.7 Discussion 98
       References 102
       Additional Readings 103

8. Why Randomization Is Essential and How to Do It 105

   Aviva Petrie

   8.1 Why We Randomize 105
   8.2 How to Randomize 108
   8.3 Discussion 111
       References 115
       Additional Readings 115

9. Statistical Inference in Clinical Trials 117

   John M. Lachin

   9.1 Introduction to Inference 117
   9.2 The Statistical Test 120
   9.3 The Importance of Sample Size 123
   9.4 Evaluation of Sample Size and Power 124
   9.5 Inference from Likelihoods 132
   9.6 Discussion 135
       References 141
       Additional Readings 142

10. Choice of Variables for Evaluation of Therapeutic Effect: The Statistical Point of View 145

    Aviva Petrie

    10.1 Scales of Measurement 145
    10.2 Response versus Concomitant Variables 146
    10.3 Reliability and Validity 147
    10.4 Objective versus Subjective Measures 148
    10.5 Multiple Variables 150
    10.6 Implications for Analysis 151
    10.7 Discussion 151
         References 153

11. Statistical Analysis of the Randomized Clinical Trial   155

John M. Lachin

    11.1   Introduction   155
    11.2   Outcome Events   156
    11.3   Prognostic Variables   160
    11.4   Mantel-Haenszel Procedure   161
    11.5   The Actuarial Life Table Method   169
    11.6   The Product Limit Method and the Log Rank Test   178
    11.7   Subgroup Analyses   181
    11.8   The Logistic Regression Model   185
    11.9   Regression Adjustment of Treatment Effects   189
    11.10   Life Table Regression Models   190
    11.11   Interim Statistical Analyses   191
            References   194

12. The Crossover Design   199

Aviva Petrie

    12.1   Introduction   199
    12.2   Discussion   202
          References   204

Part IV: IMPLEMENTATION OF THE RANDOMIZED CLINICAL TRIAL

13. Elements of an Ideal Protocol   207

Leslie J. Schoenfield

    13.1   Introduction   207
          Reference   212

14. Achieving an Adequate Sample Size: The Multicenter Trial   213

Niels Tygstrup

    14.1   Study Duration   213
    14.2   The Multicenter Trial   215
    14.3   Discussion   216
          Additional Readings   218

15. The Execution of a Protocol   219

John M. Lachin

    15.1   Organization   219
    15.2   Standardization   222

15.3 Study Forms 222
15.4 Computerization 225
15.5 Training and Pretesting 226
15.6 Quality Assessment 227
15.7 Morale 229
15.8 Discussion 230
    References 233
    Additional Readings 234

16. Early Termination of a Clinical Trial   235

    Thomas C. Chalmers

    16.1 The Decision to Stop 235
    16.2 Additional Considerations 236
    16.3 Blinding 238
    16.4 Discussion 241
        References 245
        Additional Readings 246

Part V: PERCEPTIONS OF THE RANDOMIZED CLINICAL TRIAL

17. Randomized Clinical Trials and the Producers   249

    Leslie J. Schoenfield

    17.1 Selection of Participants 249
    17.2 Testing and Training 250
    17.3 Communications 251
    17.4 Ancillary Studies and Publications 251
    17.5 Discussion 252
        Additional Readings 256

18. Randomized Clinical Trials and the Consumers   257

    Thomas C. Chalmers

    18.1 Introduction 257
    18.2 Discussion 262
        References 263

19. Randomized Clinical Trials and the Patients   265

    Povl Riis

    19.1 Ethical Considerations 265
    19.2 The Helsinki Declaration 266
    19.3 Impact of the Declaration 269
    19.4 Discussion 271
        Reference 274
        Additional Readings 275

20. Randomized Clinical Trials and the Public 277
Franz J. Ingelfinger
  20.1 Introduction 277
  20.2 Discussion 280

Part VI: APPENDIXES

A. National Institutes of Health Guidelines
  for Data-Safety Monitoring in Clinical Trials   285
     Reference 286

B. Declaration of Helsinki, II   287
     Introduction 287
  I.   Basic Principles 288
  II. Medical Research Combined with Professional
       Care (Clinical Research) 290
  III. Nontherapeutic Biomedical Research Involving
       Human Subjects (Nonclinical Biomedical Research) 291

Index   293

THE RANDOMIZED CLINICAL TRIAL AND THERAPEUTIC DECISIONS

Part I
The Relation between Clinical Medicine
and the Randomized Clinical Trial

1
How Therapeutic Decisions Are Motivated

POVL RIIS
Herlev Hospital
University of Copenhagen
Herlev, Denmark

1.1 INTRODUCTION

If clinicians are asked how therapeutic and diagnostic decisions are made, they will probably answer that it is an extremely complicated process. They may even say that the practice of medicine is an artistic process which is too complicated to understand by means of scientific methods. This of course is not true. Rather we can say that making a diagnosis is simplicity instead of complexity, and that in deciding on a treatment the situation is often lack of knowledge instead of complexity of decision.

Figure 1.1 depicts how clinicians often work. The patient contacts the physician, who then collects the history, signs, and laboratory data and compares these components with his knowledge of the clinical manifestations of different diseases. If they suit each other, he is able to make a diagnostic decision. Immediately afterward he asks himself whether this diagnosis is sufficiently certain to elicit a rational therapy. If the answer is yes, then a treatment is selected and hopefully the patient will soon thereafter be cured. We all know that this process may be completed within a very short time and in such cases it may appear that the physician is an artist at work. But in other cases the

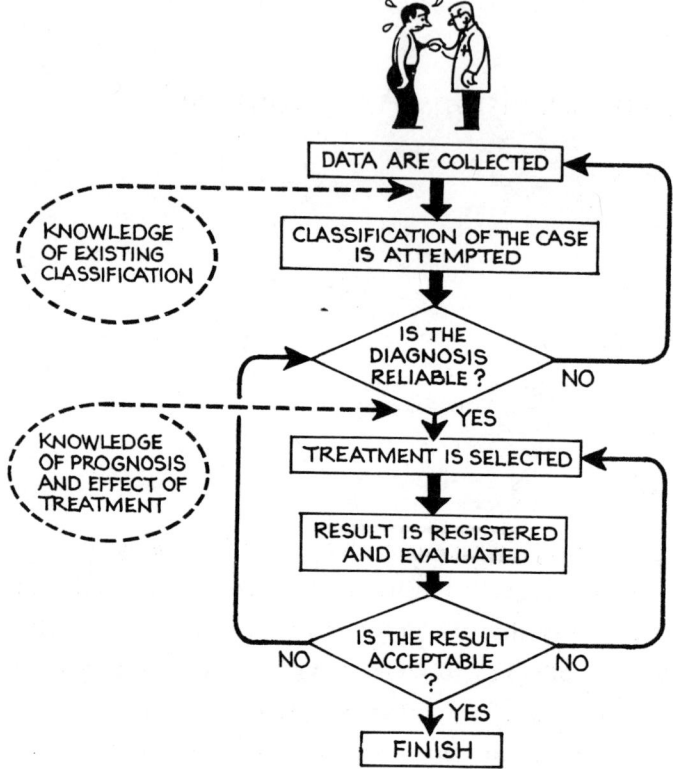

FIGURE 1.1 A flowchart of medical decision making.

process can take weeks and sometimes involve a whole medical department; and then the the patient doesn't think that his physician is an artist.

When a physician has made his diagnosis, he then asks himself: "What do we know about the different treatments in this disease?" This is the real therapeutic decision. Does the brain's store of therapeutic knowledge consist of beliefs, or is it scientific knowledge based on controlled clinical studies?

If colleagues from departments of biochemistry or physiology are asked what clinicians should do to determine the right treatment for a given condition, they may say that we should first determine all the physiochemical steps in the disease process so that we can determine how best to interrupt its progress. But we cannot wait for such a scientific revolution in the basic sciences; we have to do something in between, we still have to treat patients here and now.

Fortunately, an increasing number of clinicians today realize that scientific methods are available, one of them being the randomized clinical trial. Unfortunately, some clinicians still do not want to undertake this tedious job. They think there must be easier methods. We still encounter heads of departments and professors of medicine who start their statements in conferences by saying: "According to my experience. . . ." or "In old Professor NN's department we always did so and so. . . . "! But experience can be biased and folklore is more often than not unfounded.

Donald Mainland (1) has mentioned that there are two types of people studying therapeutics: One is the that-group, people who examine things to show that a given therapy has a certain effect; and the other is the if-group, who want to examine if a certain therapy works in a given disease. We hope to be able to recruit more members to the small if-group through this book.

It is sometimes felt that knowing the principles of the randomized clinical trial is only necessary for those who are active in clinical research. This is certainly not true. Of course, a clinical researcher who plans to work with these problems has to know the methods, but what is equally important is that all clinicians examining and treating patients should understand the main principles of the randomized clinical trial.

The half-life of clinical knowledge today is very short--8, 10, or 12 years, certainly not longer. The influx of new information from journals, meetings, and other sources is very great. A physician must constantly exchange old knowledge with new knowledge. But how do we choose and select what of this vast information is reliable? It should be on the basis of scientific principles, such as the randomized trial. Journals and other written information could be filed in one of two ways: horizontally or vertically. More physicians ought to learn to select and file information vertically, i.e., let some of it go in their wastepaper baskets, instead of horizontally on their shelves. Otherwise one will become confused by the mixture of sometimes true, sometimes false, sometimes intermediate information.

There are two basic principles of the controlled clinical trial on which I shall comment briefly. They are so simple that I should perhaps not even mention them here. The first is that all clinical judgments should be based on comparisons. A statistic such as the percentage of successes with a treatment has no value in the decision process without being <u>compared</u> to something else, compared to that observed in an appropriate control or untreated group. The second basic concept is that everything changes, everything varies. Patients' symptoms and reactions change all the time, our measurement instruments change all the time, and the clinician himself changes as an observer. This <u>variation</u> makes experiments in clinical medicine difficult but all the more necessary.

In biophysics we often use the term <u>signal-to-noise ratio</u>. In clinical medicine the "signal" consists of the patients who show a reaction which is really due to treatment, while the "noise" consists of all the patients who would have reacted regardless of whether or not they had been treated. In some cases the signal is strong and the noise weak and a simple study can establish benefit. But in many cases the signal is weak while the noise is strong and a carefully conducted design will be required to show benefit.

1.2 DISCUSSION
Decision Theory

<u>Ingelfinger</u>
Dr. Riis has described the importance of making therapeutic decisions on the basis of randomized, controlled trials. I would like to emphasize

an even greater ideal, which theoretically is possible if we had enough information.

In an issue of the <u>New England Journal of Medicine</u> were published two papers; one presented a primer on statistical models for decision making (2), while the other applied these models to therapeutic decision making (3), which is what we are talking about. To illustrate these techniques, the second article considered the question of how a physician should decide whether or not to operate in a young man with symptoms indicating possible appendicitis. To make this decision, emphasizing the theoretical ideal, the physician should know something about the probability parameters involved.

Let's say we're interested in mortality. What the physician needs to know is the likelihood (i.e., the probability) that, if the patient has this operation, he will be found to have appendicitis blast, i.e., that the physician will have made the right decision. The physician also needs to consider that if he operates and the patient does not have the disease, then there is a certain risk of mortality engendered, and it was suggested that it might be 1 out of 1000, i.e., 0.1% mortality. Likewise, a decision not to operate but with appendicitis present, these authors suggest, will yield a 4% mortality. On the basis of such figures, and the probability whether or not the patient has appendicitis, they developed formulas which should theoretically help the physician to decide whether or not to operate.

The difficulty with this approach is that we do not know the true probabilities or the true mortality rates exactly. They might be the correct values in Italy, but not in Germany or elsewhere. Futhermore, I only talked about mortality, but we are also interested in morbidity. I have not mentioned anything about other considerations such as risks and costs that would influence these decisions.

The problem then is to determine the likelihoods for the various decisions and pursuant events. There can never be enough analyzed controlled trials to provide dependable estimates. We may have to pick just a few major points such as mortality, but in the absence of such ideal decision making, I am afraid the physician will continue to base his decision on extraneous considerations.

<u>Lachin</u>
Statistical decision theory was developed to be applied to the broad class of decisions, not only to medical decisions but to decisions we all reach in everyday life. Decision theory provides a strategy so that the decision maker would optimize his potential gains over a period of time making similar decisions. There are two elements that go into the process, one is a consideration of the likelihoods of the different outcomes for the different actions that could be taken, e.g. the likelihood of mortality following the decision to operate or not to operate. The second element of the decision process is a consideration of the potential losses, or the costs of an incorrect decision. For

example, in a gamble the actions that one might take will depend largely on the size of the bet. In the long run one wants to use a system for reaching decisions so that the expected gains are maximized or the expected losses minimized. As Dr. Ingelfinger pointed out, this is an idealization; however, it has very practical implications for every decision that we make. We must learn to consider the relative likelihood of each different outcome given every action that we take, and the potential losses that are to be incurred. To adopt this approach thus requires estimates of these likelihoods, which are often best obtained through a randomized controlled trial.

Blum
The problem would be relatively simple if we had only one option, to operate or not to operate, but in most clinical situations many things may happen or not happen.

Riis
Well, even if decision theory can not solve all of the clinician's problems, a knowledge of it may be useful in stimulating his critical attitude.

Ingelfinger
Even though I said it was an unattainable ideal, at least with our present knowledge, something has been achieved if we all realize that we should carefully go through an evaluation of the possible losses and gains for each patient.

Sufficiency of the Clinical Trial

Schoenfield
Overall, I agree to the necessity of the randomized controlled trial, but we have to keep in mind that a given clinical trial may not be sufficient for all therapeutic decisions. It is conceivable but very unlikely because of the many variables that go into the selection of patients, the techniques of the investigators, the outcome measures, etc. Many clinical trials are almost always needed.

A few years back we were studying the effects of treatments in chronic active hepatitis (4). In that particular trial we established a particular definition for chronic active hepatitis, but this was not the total spectrum of the disease. It showed that steroid was clearly superior to placebo and to azathioprine in this group of patients, but not necessarily in all patients with chronic active hepatitis. It is important as we read the reports of clinical trials to understand the population that was studied. The trial may have employed a restricted population so that the results turn out not to be sufficient for clinical use.

Tygstrup
The randomized clinical trial will never answer all the questions about the therapeutic use of a new agent. For example, it cannot be expected

that it will disclose the rare toxic reactions which would require thousands of patients under study.

Wright
A classic example is the halothane controversy. It was passionately felt by anaesthesiologists that this was the safest anaesthetic available because there were no hepatotoxic effects in animals. They refuted the view of hepatologists that a small group of patients would develop liver damage--sometimes fatal--from halothane. This is precisely what was demonstrated, however, in subsequent large-scale studies (5). Randomized controlled trials should be started as early as possible, therefore, to evaluate both efficacy and adverse reactions.

Having said this, it should also be stressed that there are limitations to such trials when they are not conducted under the conditions which will exist when the therapy is used in clinical practice. To avoid this we in the United Kingdom try particularly to conduct trials in the community among general practitioners. As an example, several early trials showed that carbenoxolone was effective in the treatment of gastric ulcer (6), but it was only when the drug was used on a large scale among general practioners that the severity of hypertension as a side effect became obvious.

Another example is the use of corticosteroids in ulcerative colitis. Many were convinced of its effectiveness, but in general practice many mild cases were overtreated, resulting in serious side effects.

The randomized controlled trial is of course very important, but it is also important that the results be applicable to the overall practice of medicine.

Lachin
Virtually all new drugs go through a variety of stages of clinical testing. The first clinical trials are conducted to evaluate gross toxicity, usually in normal volunteers. The next phase then evaluates the efficacy of the drug in the treatment of the target disease. At this stage certain exclusions are usually introduced, such as females capable of bearing children because of the possible teratogenic effects. This is then followed by larger-scale studies of the safety of the drug, but again in selected patient populations. At that point if the drug has been shown to be safe and effective, it may be marketed.

What does the physician do, however, when he wishes to prescribe the agent to a female of child-bearing potential? Package inserts may help, but often these simply state that certain types of patients, such as young females, have not been studied. There are no simple solutions to such problems. The best approach available appears to be to continue to collect data after a drug goes into widespread use. Based on a given patient's characteristics, a decision might be made as to whether or not to prescribe the agent. Having done so, the physician then has a responsibility to record the outcome, because such patients may respond very differently from those studied in the clinical trials. If an unexpected response to the drug does occur, I think it is then the physician's responsibility to communicate the finding to the medical community. Information--especially scientific information--is of no value until it is communicated.

Schoenfield
Another important facet in decision making which should not be forgotten is the influence of tradition and folklore. Well-known examples are the high-residue diet in diverticulosis and intolerance to fried and fatty foods in gallstones. When we talk about the significance of the randomized controlled trial, its role in evaluating traditions should also be borne in mind.

Tygstrup
We have learned that our decision making could be much improved by better data, by estimates of probabilities. But these estimates sometimes come from very incomplete and often biased data, what we call "experience" and "'clinical impressions," traditional thinking, and ill-founded belief in authorities. The human brain is said to be an excellent analytical machine, but a bad memory machine. The opposite is the case of the computer, and if we could feed good data into the computer, our decision making could be improved. Good data are what we should get from the randomized controlled trial.

REFERENCES

1. Mainland, D., Elementary Medical Statistics, Saunders, Philadelphia and London, 1964.
2. McNeil, B. J., Keeler, E., and Adelstein, S. J., Primer on certain elements of medical decision making, N. Engl. J. Med., 1975, 293, 212-215.
3. Pauker, S. G., and Kassirer, J. P., Therapeutic decision making: A cost-benefit analysis, N. Engl. J. Med., 1975, 293, 229-234.
4. Soloway, R. D., Summerskill, W. H. J., Baggenstoss, A. H , Geal, M. G., Gitnick, G. L., Elveback, L. R., and Schoenfield, L. J., Clinical, biochemical, and histological remission of severe chronic active liver disease: A controlled study of treatments and early prognosis, Gastroenterology, 1972, 63, 820-833.
5. Wright, R., Eade, O. E., Chisholm, M., Hawksley, M., Lloyd, B., Moles, T. M., Edwards, J. C., and Gardner, M. J., Controlled prospective study of the effect on liver function of multiple exposures to halothane, Lancet, 1975, i, 817.
6. Doll, R., Hill, I. D., Hutton, C., and Underwood, D. J., Clinical trial of a triterpenoid liquorice compound in gastric ulcer and duodenal ulcer, Lancet, 1962, ii, 793.

ADDITIONAL READINGS

Birnbaum, A., and Maxwell, A. E., Classification procedures based on Bayes' formula, Appl. Stat., 1960, 9, 152-169.

Feinstein, A., Clinical Judgment, Williams & Wilkins, Baltimore, 1967.

Food and Drug Administration, General Considerations for the Clinical Evaluation of Drugs, FDA publication 77-3040, U.S. Government Printing Office, 1977.

Galen, R. S., and Gambino, S. R., Beyond Normality: The Predictive Value and Efficiency of Medical Diagnosis, Wiley, New York, 1975.

Jick, H., The discovery of drug-induced illness, N. Engl. J. Med., 1977, 296, 481-485.

Ledley, R. S. and Lusted, L. B., Reasoning foundations of medical diagnosis, Science, 1959, 130, 9-12.

Lusted, L., Introduction to Medical Decision Making, Thomas, Springfield, Ill., 1968.

Wulff, H., Rational Diagnosis and Treatment, Blackwell, Oxford, 1976.

2
The Randomized Clinical Trial as a Basis for Therapeutic Decisions

THOMAS C. CHALMERS
The Mount Sinai Medical Center
Mount Sinai School of Medicine
New York, New York

2.1 INTRODUCTION

I have made many mistakes in my life practicing medicine. A major one was my acceptance of a trial in cirrhosis comparing high-protein diets with a <u>nonrandomized</u> control group (1). It was on this basis that many of us began to treat cirrhotic patients with a high-protein diet. When the patients went into coma we put a tube down into their stomachs to give them the diet homogenized. When they died in coma, we said that we must not have given them enough.

Another example is a study done by a surgeon in Boston who showed favorable results when he shunted patients with cirrhosis while the control group had a markedly worse survival (2). But they were <u>historical</u> controls. It was claimed that he operated on the patients with a good prognosis and not on those with a poor prognosis. He has said that was wrong, he never selected his patients, he only selected the time at which he conducted the operation. In other words he operated on everybody who lived long enough to get into good enough shape for surgery, and he compared these with a group of patients that included some who did not live long enough to get into good enough shape for surgery.

These are just two of the many studies which have led me to become an advocate of the randomized, controlled clinical trial. Randomization alone is worthless without adequate controls and adequate blinding of controls. Likewise, the use of nonrandomized controls is hazardous. We have to keep in mind that randomization not only eliminates bias in treatment assignment, it provides for an unbiased comparison between the groups no matter how the patients are selected for study.

Another example which convinced me that more randomized, controlled clinical trials were needed was my experience treating patients with gastrointestinal hemorrhage. A young man came into the hospital who had a massive hemorrhage and who later died without surgery. The next young man admitted with massive hemorrhage was operated on earlier than he might have been if the previous patient had not died without surgery, and he did well. The next slightly older man was operated on and he also did well. The next still older man was operated on and he did well. Then a patient was operated on and died. The next patient had surgery much later than he would have if the previous patient had not died.

Decision making is a flowing thing. The difference between a skilled older clinician and a young physician who is learning is that the young are overly impressed by the last patient they saw. When one is older he has forgotten the patient he saw yesterday! This gives the older doctor the clinical judgment we would all have if we based our decisions on large experiences in the past and on randomized clinical trials, rather than on one or two recent events in highly variable patients.

The randomized clinical has been criticized as a decision making technique for many reasons, but usually they add up to criticisms of poorly conceived studies. One clinical trial done well in a highly selected group of patients is entirely sufficient to learn how to treat a highly selected group of patients. But such a trial is not sufficient to learn how to best treat a broader group of patients who may be very much unlike the ones included in that trial. We need to emphasize that there never has been a universally applicable clinical trial. All have problems because they are carried out in variably selected patients. We often need several trials to detect the exact risk/benefit ratio of a given new therapy compared with the old, in many different kinds of patients.

One hears computer medicine criticized because of the GIGO principle (garbage in, garbage out). What the critics forget is that the clinician at the bedside may be gathering the same old garbage and he is therefore going to get the same old garbage out.

2.2   DISCUSSION
Controls and Trial Validity

Schoenfield
To support this point further it should be emphasized that about 80% of the uncontrolled trials reported in the literature showed that the treatment was effective, whereas only 25% of the randomized controlled trials showed the treatments evaluated to be effective (3). It makes quite a difference whether or not the trial is controlled.

Chalmers
As a further example, consider the results in Table 2.1 of the therapeutic trials for portacaval shunting (Adapted from 4). In articles with adequate controls, none reveal marked enthusiasm, 3 reveal moderate, and 5 no enthusiasm for the procedure, while 76 of the 99 articles with poor or no controls show marked enthusiasm. The difference between the controlled and uncontrolled trials is highly significant and shows that the best way to get a positive result is to leave out the controls.

Other Factors--Blinding

Petrie
It should be pointed out, however, that randomization and controls alone may not be sufficient to insure that the conlusions are valid. The other aspects of the trial which might also allow bias to affect the conclusions cannot be neglected.

TABLE 2.1 Conclusions versus Validity of Controls in Clinical Trials of Portacaval Shunting

Controls	Degree of enthusiam			Total
	Marked	Moderate	None	
Adequate	0	3	5	8
Poor	18	3	2	23
None	58	15	3	76

Source: Adapted from Ref. 4. Reprinted by permission from Chalmers, T. C., Randomized controlled clinical trials in diseases of the liver, in Progress In Liver Diseases, Volume V, (H. Popper and F. Schaffner, eds.), Grune & Stratton, New York, 1976, pp. 450-455.

Chalmers

Among the most important of these considerations is blinding. If the physician knows which therapy each patient is receiving, i.e., if the trial is not blinded, and if the physician has a bias as to which therapy is better, he may be inclined to prescribe additional ancillary therapies to the patients receiving the therapy he doesn't favor. The effects of randomization are then destroyed since in effect the favored treatment group is compared to a group receiving the control therapy plus various ancillary therapies.

The physician may also distort the study by withdrawal of some patients and not of others. Randomization does no good if chance determines which therapy each patient receives and then bias is allowed to determine which patients are withdrawn. Randomization also does no good if the physician is able to recognize which treatment appears to be better and then stops the study when it looks like the treatment that is better happens to be the one he believes in.

Justifications for Controls

Juhl

Although the randomized, controlled trial is undoubtedly valuable, I feel we must also consider when a clinical trial is justified. Figure 2.1 exemplifies the situation in the case of four different liver diseases and four different treatments (from 5). There is a prognostic spectrum

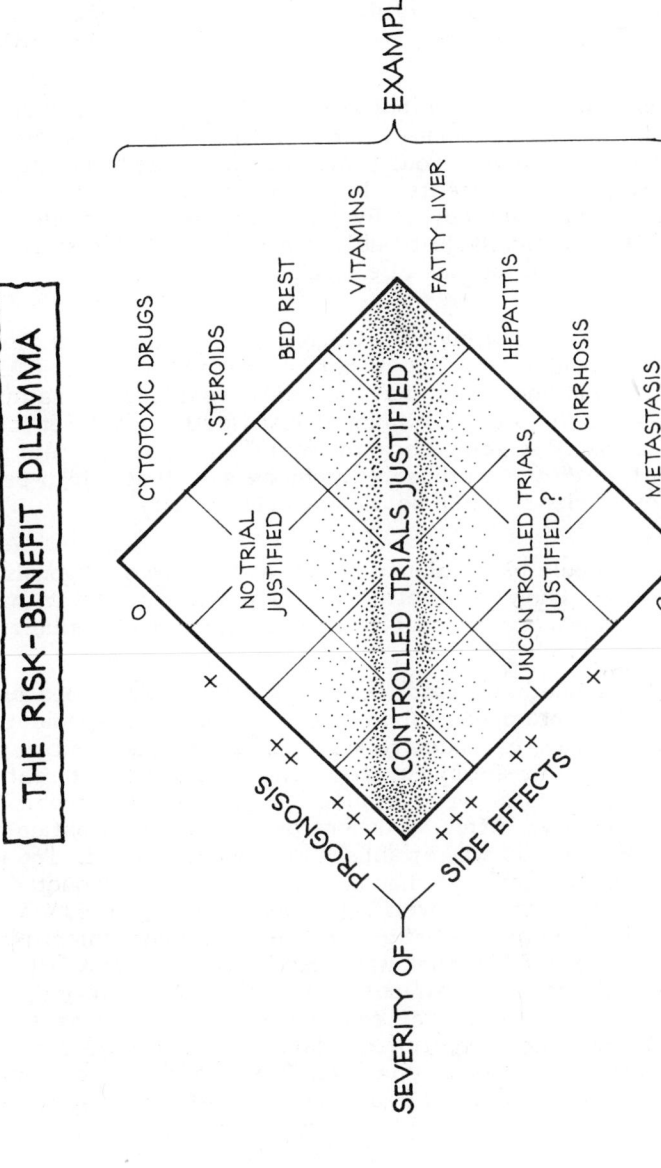

FIGURE 2.1 Prognosis versus side effects of treatment and the justification of controlled trials. (From Ref. 5.)

from fatty liver to liver metastases, and a spectrum of therapies, from vitamin therapy to cytotoxic drugs, with increasing risk and severity of associated side effects. The fatty liver has a very good prognosis, liver metastases a very bad prognosis, and in between there are hepatitis and cirrhosis.

There has to be a balance between possible benefits and risks of treatment. In the upper part of the diamond there is no balance, because a disease with a very good prognosis should not be treated with a drug with severe side effects. In the lower part of the diamond exemplified by vitamin therapy of liver metastases, uncontrolled trials may be considered ethically justifiable due to lack of side effects but probably not very useful for lack of efficacy.

Ingelfinger
Isn't this figure based on prejudice? Uncontrolled data is being inserted as the basis for deciding whether or not controlled trials are justified. As an example you indicated that vitamins would do no harm; the implication is that the use of vitamins is justified for whatever disease you wish to study. But going back to what Tom Chalmers said about using high-protein diets, it probably might be said that a high-protein diet in liver insufficiency would not do any harm either.

Juhl
I agree. There should be a balance between the known prognosis of a disease against the known side effects of a treatment, and it may be impossible to obtain this knowledge without using controlled studies.

Blum
As an example of unethical practices in clinical research, Beecher (6) cited studies of chloramphenicol in the treatment of typhoid fever. Around 1950, a series of uncontrolled studies had demonstrated the favorable effect of this antibiotic on a dangerous and life-threatening disease. The effect was so overwhelming that a controlled, double-blind study was unnecessary. After an uncontrolled study in 10 patients the effect of chloramphenicol was established beyond any doubt. Ten years later a double-blind, randomized, controlled trial was conducted with chloramphenicol in typhoid fever. It was shown that 23% of the placebo-treated patients and 8% of the chloramphenicol-treated patients died. This clinical trial was unecessary and highly unethical. Once the effect of a treatment has been demonstrated, it is inappropriate to perform a trial comparing it with a less effective treatment. Randomized, controlled trials should only be performed when there is a real therapeutic dilemma. The physician who conducted the clinical trial with chloramphenicol already knew that chloramphenicol was better than placebo in typhoid fever.

Lachin
I disagree. In my opinion the ethics relate not to the conduct of the controlled trial, but rather to the initial conduct of an uncontrolled

trial. In such cases the controlled trial is scientifically necessary to evaluate the therapy. There have been far too many instances of therapies shown to be effective in uncontrolled experience but shown to be ineffective or even harmful in a later controlled trial. If a controlled trial had been done initially, those lives might have been spared.

I would like to become a little philosophical at this point. We have been talking about the use of the randomized, controlled trial as necessary and sufficient for medical decision making. We have heard arguments against clinical trials as being neither necessary nor justified in some situations and others in favor of uncontrolled trials. The randomized, controlled trial, however, is the essence of a scientific approach in medicine. Science is a very human enterprise; it is inherently imperfect. Science is nothing more than a set of principles which are intended to minimize the uncertainty with which decisions are made. Science and the randomized, controlled trial do not guarantee correct decisions, but they are such that in the long run, such decisions will be accurate more often than not.

REFERENCES

1. Patek, A. J., Post, J., Ratnoff, O. D., Mankin, H. and Hillman, R. W., Dietary treatment of cirrhosis, J. Am. Med. Assoc., 1948, 138, 543-550.

2. Linton, R. R., Portacaval shunts in the treatment of portal hypertension; with special reference on patients previously operated upon, N. Engl. J. Med., 1948, 238, 723-727.

3. Foulds, G. A., Clinical Research in psychiatry, J. Ment. Sci., 1958, 104, 259.

4. Chalmers, T. C., Randomized controlled clinical trials in diseases of the liver, in Progress In Liver Diseases, Volume V, (H. Popper and F. Schaffner, eds.), Grune & Stratton, New York, 1976, pp. 450-455.

5. Tygstrup, N., and Juhl, E., Dilemmas of controlled clinical trials in hepatology, in The Liver and Its Diseases , (F. Schaffner, S. Sherlock, and C. M. Leevy, eds.), Intercontinental Medical Book Corporation, New York, 1974, pp. 64-75.

6. Beecher, H. K., Ethics and clinical research, N. Engl. J. Med., 1966, 274, 354-360.

ADDITIONAL READINGS

Gehan, E. A., and Freireich, E. J., Non-randomized controls in cancer clinical trials, N. Engl. J. Med., 1974, 290, 198-203.

Weinstein, M. C., Allocation of subjects in medical experiments, N. Engl. J. Med., 1974, 291, 1278-1285.

Byar, D. P., Simon, R. M., Friedewald, W. T., Schlesselman, J. J., DeMets, D. L., Ellenberg, J. H., Gail, M. H., and Ware, J. H., Randomized clinical trials--Perspectives on some recent ideas., N. Engl. J. Med., 1976, 295, 74-80.

3
Contributions of Randomized Clinical Trials over a Decade (1964–1973) to Gastroenterological Therapy

ERIK JUHL
Hvidovre Hospital
University of Copenhagen
Copenhagen, Denmark

3.1 INTRODUCTION

In 1964 Truelove and Wright (1) published a survey of controlled therapeutic trials. In conclusion they declared: "We judge that the need for controlled therapeutic trials will multiply rather than dwindle as scientific inquiry into disease develops." We later tested this forecast and reviewed the literature to investigate the rate at which the randomized, controlled clinical trial been used in gastroenterology during the decade 1964-1973 (2, 3).

A clinical trial was defined as a study where patients were allocated to a treatment and a control group at random, and where the therapeutic effects were evaluated on the basis of the clinically relevant outcome, e.g., complete ulcer healing, and not on the basis of pure laboratory data, e.g., maximum acidity output or the level of aminotransferases.

The MEDLARS facility was employed to search for any trial which studied the effects of drug therapy, radiotherapy, surgery, or other types of therapy in the treatment of digestive diseases in man. Key words such as comparative study and clinical research were used in the search because they should apply to reports of clinical trials according to the existing MEDLARS instructions. The outcome of the search was 1590 reference citations. After careful study of all reports, except for 25 that were not available, only 306 trials were found to fulfill our criteria described above. These papers form the basis of the following presentation.

During the 10-year period 1964-1973, 32,911 articles concerning therapy in gastroenterology have been recorded in MEDLARS and less than 1% fulfilled the criteria of a randomized controlled trial! Clinical trials were used most commonly in the evaluation of drugs (4%), less commonly with surgical procedures (1%). Figure 3.1 shows the change in the rate with which clinical trials were used during this decade. In

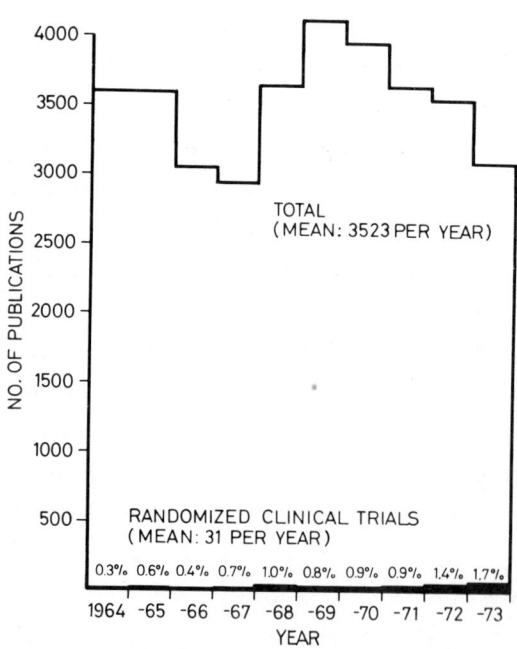

FIGURE 3.1 Number of citations in MEDLARS regarding therapies in gastroenterology during the decade 1964-1974. The frequency of clinical trials among these citations is recorded for each year. (From Ref. 2. Reprinted by permission of the N. Engl. J. Med., 1977, 296, 20-22.)

1964, 0.4% of the studies on treatment in gastroenterology were randomized controlled trials; by 1973 this had increased to 1.8%, a statistically significant increase though, in my opinion, far from the figure anticipated by Truelove and Wright.

Table 3.1 lists the 10 leading countries from which the 306 clinical trials originated. Eighty percent of the 306 trials were carried out in these 10 countries; Great Britain and the United Sataes account for about half the trials. Great Britain also accounts for the largest number of medical journals having published clinical trials in gastroenterology, there being 6 British, 3 North American, and 1 Scandinavian journal. Almost half the clinical trials appeared in these 10 journals.

Approximately one-quarter (23%) of the studies were multicenter, mostly with only two collaborating units. Several of these multicenter studies were carried out in general practice, mostly by British general practitioners. Only 8 were multinational, and 4 binational (Figure 3.2). Table 3.2 shows that the period of observation was remarkably short in

TABLE 3.1 Leading Countries of Origin of Randomized Controlled Trials

Country	Published clinical trials	
	Number	Percent
Great Britain	83	27
United States	75	25
Italy	16	5
West Germany	15	5
Japan	13	4
Denmark	11	4
South Africa	10	3
Australia	9	3
France	7	2
Norway	7	2
Total	246	80

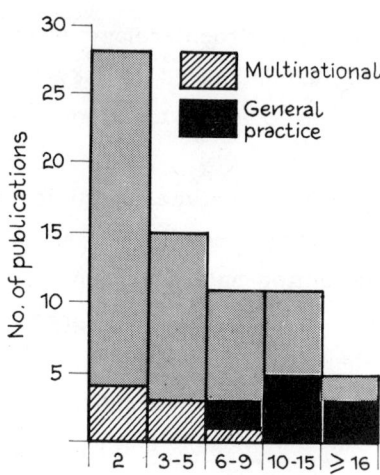

FIGURE 3.2 Characteristics of published clinical trials.

many trials; in 25% it covered less than two weeks and in only 13% did it exceed one year.

The disease most commonly studied was duodenal ulcer, which is now explored in greater detail.

According to most textbooks of internal medicine, nonsurgical treatment of duodenal ulcer implied, in 1964, the use of anticholinergics, antacids, diet, rest, and sedatives (Table 3.3). But

TABLE 3.2 Period of Observation in the Published Clinical Trials

Period	Number of publications	Cumulated percent
Less than 2 weeks	84	28
2-4 weeks	47	44
1-2 months	88	73
3-12 months	42	87
1-2 years	26	96
More than 2 years	13	100
No information provided	6	

TABLE 3.3 Nonoperative Treatment of Duodenal Ulcer

Treatment	Treatment used in		Effect documented by RCT		No effect documented by RCT		RCT	
	1964	1973	Before 1964	1964-73	Before 1964	1964-73	Before 1964	1964-73
Anticholinergics	+	+			+	+		
Antacids	+	+				+	+	
Diet	+	+			+			+
Bedrest	+	(+)		+				
Sedatives	+	(+)		+	+			
Carbenoxolone	0	0					+	
Antipeptics	0	0	+					
Stilbestrol	0	0				+	+	+
Gastric freezing	0	0						

according to Truelove and Wright, only therapy with stilbestrol was documented by a clinical trial to promote healing of the ulcer (specifically in men with an ulcer history of less than 10 years). They noted that in 1964, clinical trials had failed to document any effect for anticholinergics, diet, sedatives, or carbenoxolone on the healing of duodenal ulcer, and clinical trials had not been performed to evaluate the effect of antacids and bedrest.

We then evaluated whether randomized controlled trials performed during the 10-year period 1964-1973 had contributed to improved treatment of duodenal ulcer and if so, to what extent. The treatment of duocenal ulcer was the subject of 57 clinical trials during the period 1964-1973. The criteria for the selection of patients participating in the trials varied greatly. Therefore, the five additional assessment criteria shown in Table 3.4 were established; only those trials fulfilling these criteria were included in the final analyses. By this means 17 trials were eliminated.

Eleven of the remaining 40 clinical trials were aimed at an evaluation of the value of anticholinergics in the treatment of duodenal

TABLE 3.4 Criteria for Review of Clinical Trials on Treatment of Duodenal Ulcer

1. Description of the patients included (age, length of history, sex ratio)

2. Differentiation between duodenal and gastric ulcer

3. Verification of a duodenal ulcer by radiography, endoscopy, or at operation

4. Treatment or follow-up period of at least 4 weeks

5. Results given as percent of patients showing a defined response per number of patients being treated

ulcer. In 8 trials the effect was compared with that of placebo. Two were positive, i.e., the difference was found to be statistically significant, and 6 were negative. Among the 3 remaining clinical trials, all negative, one used antacid as a a control group, one another anticholinergic, and one a higher dose of the same anticholinergic.

Figure 3.3 illustrates the cumulative net cure rate of anticholinergics defined as the cure rate in the treatment group minus the cure rate in the control group. Cure rate is the percentage of patients responding to treatment. Initially, the clinical cure rate after anticholinergics was 56%; however, as trials increased in number, the cumulative clinical cure rate declined, approaching zero. The cumulative radiological cure rate has not at any time been significantly different from zero. During the same a period of time, however,

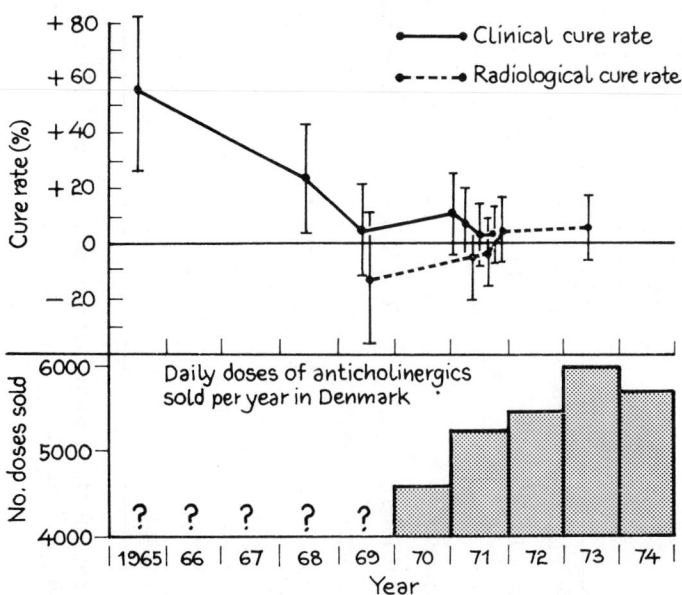

FIGURE 3.3 Cumulative difference in the cure rate of anticholinergics versus that of controls in the treatment of duodenal ulcer, ±SE of the difference. (Data from Ref. 3.)

TABLE 3.5 Recommendations in Textbooks for Nonsurgical Treatment of Duodenal Ulcer Compared with Results of Randomized Clinical Trials during 1964-1974

	Result of clinical trials before 1964	Recommendation in textbooks for treatment in 1964	Result of clinical trials 1964-1974	Recommendation in textbooks for treatment in 1974
Anticholinergics	No effect	Recommended	No effect	Recommended
Antacids	No trials	Recommended	No effect	Recommended
Diet	No effect	Recommended	No RCT	? Recommended[a]
Bedrest	No trials	Recommended	No RCT	? Recommended
Sedatives	No effect	Recommended	No RCT	? Recommended
Giving up smoking	No trials	Recommended	No RCT	Recommended
Carbenoxolone	No effect	Not recommended	Effect	Not recommended
Estrogens	Effect	Not recommended	No effect	Not recommended
Deglycyrrhizinated liquorice	No trials		No effect	Not recommended
Antipeptics	No trials		Effect	Not recommended

[a]Treatment recommended in some textbooks but not in other textbooks.
Source: Ref. 3.

despite the preponderance of negative studies, there was an increasing consumption of anticholinergic drugs, at least in Denmark.

In the same way, clinical trials of carbenoxolone, antacids, antipeptics, gastric freezing, diet, bedrest, sedatives, stilbestrol, and giving up smoking were investigated and the impact of these trials during 1964-1973 is shown in Table 3.5. The two types of therapy (anticholinergics and antacids) which were documented during the interval 1964-1973 to be without effect are--according to textbooks in 1974--nonetheless still in general use in most countries. Trials aimed at an evaluation of four of the treatments most commonly used in cases of duodenal ulcer (diet, bedrest, sedatives, giving up smoking) have not been performed, and the only two types of treatments documented to be effective (carbenoxolone and antipeptics) were not in general use.

We conclude, therefore, that clinical trials aimed at an evaluation of the treatments of duodenal ulcer were not only few in number during the examined period, but that the impact of clinical trials in this field had also been very small. Since 1974, however, new trials and new therapies (e.g., cimetidine) have been studied which have changed the therapeutic spectrum.

3.2 DISCUSSION

Riis
We have seen an example of how much is lacking in our file of experience, and I will comment on the consequences for clinical medicine. As of 1974, only a few studies had demonstrated successful treatment of duodenal ulcer without surgery, and a number of others produced negative results. Thus, in my department in 1974 we did not consider any medical treatment of duodenal ulcer effective. We could have tried to guess which medical therapies might have worked and then hoped for the best, but by following these results strictly, i.e., omitting medical treatment, we saved a lot of time and money for our patients. It is a problem of large consequences for the medical care system.

Schoenfield
What the randomized trial had contributed to gastroentrology in this decade is perhaps a bit discouraging. We had all hoped for more, and what we should try to do now is perhaps to understand why our

expectations were not reached. Either the randomized clinical trial has had some limitations in its design, or perhaps we have taken the data from clinical trials and generalized the results beyond the scope of the populations studied.

REFERENCES

1. Truelove, S. C., and Wright, R., The controlled therapeutic trial in gastroenterology, Amer. J. Dig. Dis., 1964, 9, 1-30.
2. Juhl, E., Christensen, E., and Tygstrup, N., The epidemiology of the gastrointestinal randomized clinical trial, N. Engl. J. Med., 1977, 296, 20-22.
3. Christensen, E., Juhl, E., and Tygstrup, N., Treatment of duodenal ulcer: Randomized clinical trials of a decade, Gastroenterology, 1977, 73, 1170-1178.

ADDITIONAL READING

Fletcher, R. H., and Fletcher, S. W., Clinical research in general medical journals: A 30-year perspective, N. Engl. J. Med., 1979, 301, 180-183.

Part II
Clinical Fundamentals of the Randomized Clinical Trial

4
Clinical Elements of the Randomized Clinical Trial

ERIK JUHL
Hvidovre Hospital
University of Copenhagen
Copenhagen, Denmark

A randomized, controlled clinical trial contains four main elements: the selection of patients for the trial, the random allocation of treatments to patients, the treatment period, and the statistical analysis. There is a very intimate connection between these four elements, and both clinical and statistical aspects are involved in each. In this and the following two chapters we shall deal with those aspects which mainly involve the physician participants in a clinical trial, and as an introduction this chapter will briefly review each of these four elements. The subsequent chapters in this part expand upon the clinical aspects of patient selection and the evaluation of success.

4.1 PATIENT SELECTION

Before admission into a trial each patient should fulfill all of the adopted entry criteria (e.g., biopsy-verified cirrhosis) and none of the criteria for exclusion should apply (e.g., pregnancy, incooperability). Patients who fail to fulfill these criteria for admission are ineligible or excluded. All admission criteria should be elaborated in such a way that it is possible to precisely characterize the types of patients studied because the results are in principle applicable only to those classes of patients.

If the admission criteria (i.e., entry minus exclusion) are comprehensive (e.g., all cases of cirrhosis), the results may be easy to apply in clinical practice, but it may be more difficult to reach a statistically significant result because the population studied is not homogeneous, and as a result the difference between treatments may be small. On the other hand, restrictive criteria (e.g., nonalcoholic cirrhosis with aminotransferase and gammaglobulin more than two times normal limits) will provide results which are less useful because they apply only to a small segment of the patient population. On the other hand, it may be easier to reach statistical significance because the more homogeneous population may yield a larger difference between treatments. These considerations will also be influenced by the number of potential trial patients, because the results of a clinical trial also depend on a sufficient number of patients.

4.2 RANDOM ALLOCATION

Randomization

Randomization is essential for the statistical analysis of a clinical trial, and therefore for the conclusions which can be drawn. Randomization helps to ensure that comparable groups are formed, not only according to recognized variables, but also with respect to unknown relevant variables. It is desirable that <u>all</u> patients fulfilling the admission criteria be randomized (with consent), and it is essential that <u>all</u> patients randomized to receive one or the other treatment be included in the final analysis of the trial. Therefore, the admission, randomization, and start of treatment should be performed immediately after each other and in the sequence mentioned.

Randomization should be conducted in such a way that the results of randomization are unpredictable and supervisible. Therefore the so-called open randomization plans, such as using the day of birth or time of admission to determine treatment allocations, do not fulfill the requirement for unpredictability, and tossing a coin at bedside does not fulfill the criterion of supervisibility.

Stratification

A related issue is stratification, which refers to the subdivision of the patients into prognostic groups often termed subgroups or <u>strata</u> (e.g., females, males). This procedure can be employed in two different situations: <u>prospective stratification</u> (prerandomization stratification), and <u>retrospective stratification</u> (postrandomization stratification) in the stastistical analysis of subgroups. Under prospective stratification the patients are subdivided into different strata and randomization is performed within each strata. This ensures homogeneity between the treatment groups on the stratified factors. Retrospective stratification in statistical analysis of the results may later be used to examine subgroups with different treatment response or to adjust for any imbalances between the groups on prognostic factors.

4.3 TREATMENT PERIOD
Experimental Design

The treatment schedule depends on the experimental design of the trial. There are three fundamental experimental designs: the group comparison, the matched pairs, and the crossover trial. In the <u>group comparison trial</u> different treatments are given simultaneously to two or more independent groups of patients, with the various treatments assigned to each patient via randomization. In the <u>matched pairs trial</u>, pairs of patients identical with respect to all relevant factors are the unit of study: one patient receives one treatment and the other receives the other treatment, both treatments assigned by randomization. In the <u>crossover trial</u> each patient receives both treatments, first treatment A (or B, depending on the results of randomization), and after a withdrawal interval, treatment B (or A).

Each design has advantages and disadvantages, and the choice depends on the nature of the clinical problem, the expected therapeutic effect, and the planned statistical analysis. The group comparison trial is the most general and universally applicable procedure. The crossover trial is only applicable in acute conditions with an almost immediate therapeutic effect which also dissipates rapidly. The withdrawal interval must be long enough for complete dissipation of the effects of the therapy. Finally, the matched pairs analysis is also most applicable to acute conditions, providing the entire patient pool can be characterized and matched pairs constructed prior to randomization. A pair, however, need not consist of two patients. One area of study ideally suited to the matched pairs design is ophthalmology, wherein a patient with two equivalent eyes is studied, one of two treatments being assigned at random to each eye.

Control Group

The control group (or reference group) for a new treatment under study should be the established treatment, provided that its therapeutic effects have been well documented. In the absence of such a standard therapy, a placebo control group should be employed.

The control group also provides a correction for the psychological effects of treatment when used in conjunction with blinding (i.e., masking) each patient to the therapy, (a single-blind study). If the doctors also are blinded to the patient's therapy in order to avoid observer bias, it is called a double-blind study.

Study Exits

During the treatment period there may be two distinct categories of patients who exit from the trial prematurely: those who are deliberately withdrawn (the withdrawals; e.g., due to drug side effects), and those who are not deliberately lost during follow-up (the dropouts; e.g., due to incooperability). In both cases bias can be introduced, and a good clinical trial is characterized by a low (and stated) number of missing patients.

4.4 STATISTICAL ANALYSIS

When the final statistical analyses are performed, many important clinical and statistical elements are involved. The first consideration is to specify the outcome measurements of therapeutic effects. The equivalence of the treatments is then tested by examining whether the observed differences between the groups could have arisen by chance when in fact the samples were derived from identical populations, as would be the case when the medical treatments studied have equivalent effects upon the variables examined. This is evaluated by conducting a statistical test which results in a p-value. For example, a value $p \leq 0.05$ means in effect that the probability of a false positive result, of claiming that a difference exists when in reality it does not, is not greater than 0.05. This probability is usually referred to as the type I error α. If the statistical test yields a nonsignificant result, when in fact there is a real difference between the treatment groups, a type II error with probability β is committed. While the α level or p-value is obtained directly from the statistical results, the β error depends on a variety of factors, most importantly sample size.

Consideration should be given to the type II error before start of the trial, that is, the investigator should decide the risk (probability) he or she is willing to take to miss a certain difference, the minimal, relevant clinical difference. This is done by considering the power of the test $1 - \beta$, i.e., the probability that a real difference (of some stated magnitude) between the groups will be shown to be significant on application of the appropriate statistical test.

If the minimal, relevant clinical difference and the type I and II errors are stated, it is possible to calculate the approximate sample size necessary to ensure the success of the trial. The sample size will be a function on the stated type I and II error levels, α and β, the desired clinical difference Δ and the variability of the outcome measurements, all but the latter being under the control of the investigators. Although the sample size calculations are a statistical exercise, the clinical investigator specifies α, β, and Δ.

If a significant difference is established (i.e., $p \leq 0.05$, the type I error), it is then necessary to measure, by an <u>estimation procedure</u> such as a confidence interval, the size of this effect and its standard error, and to consider whether it is of clinical importance. On the other hand, if no statistically significant difference is found between the two treatment groups, it is then necessary to calulate the probability β of having missed a difference of a given magnitude.

These then are some of the basic considerations of importance to clinicians in the design of a clinical trial. All are discussed in greater detail in subsequent chapters.

4.5 DISCUSSION
Choice of Type I and Type II Errors

<u>Tygstrup</u>
The message is that the clinician should carefully consider which levels of α and β are relevant from a clinical point of view for a particular clinical trial. The choice of α and β in a clinical trial is not a problem for the statistician, it is a problem for the clinician, and the acceptable risks of a false positive (α) or a false negative (β) result may vary widely from one trial to another.

This process is related to a consideration of the risk-benefit dilemma discussed previously by Dr. Juhl (Figure 2.1). For example, if an investigator believes that a serious disease may be relieved by a relatively harmless agent, he may be unwilling to accept a false negative result, and therefore β should be small. If there is no alternative therapy available, a false positive result may not be too bothersome and he might then choose an α level greater than the conventional 0.05.

<u>Lachin</u>
Obviously, α and β should depend on the clinician's sense of loss to be incurred if we were to make either of these errors. The greater the potential consequences, the smaller α and β should be. The problem, however, is that as either α or β gets smaller, the required sample size increases. Often the target sample size is based on the number of available patients which may be difficult to increase. In this case, if β is too large, the only recourse is to increase α in order to decrease β.

<u>Tygstrup</u>
If the desired β cannot be obtained with the number of patients expected to be obtained, then perhaps consideration should be given to dropping the trial or conducting a multicenter trial.

Clinical Elements   39

Lachin
The National Cooperative Gallstone Study (NCGS) (1) illustrates these problems. The NCGS had two objectives: to assess the efficacy and the safety of chenodeoxycholic acid in the dissolution of cholesterol gallstones. A relatively good alternative treatment is available, namely, surgery. Gallbladder removal is considered minor surgery, but though it is relatively safe there are still potential risks involved. With this in mind, a relatively small α level was used in evaluating efficacy, $\alpha = 0.01$. Considering toxicity, however, which would entail the greater loss: making a type I error, i.e., falsely rejecting the null hypothesis, or making a type II error, i.e., failing to detect true toxicity? In light of the potential hepatotoxicity of the agent, it was felt that the loss entailed by a type I error was not very great, but we wanted to be sure to reject the null hypothesis if the treatment did cause significant toxicity. Therefore, a larger α, ($\alpha = 0.05$) was employed in order to reduce β with the sample size chosen.

Clinical Significance

Student
Is clinical significance a subjective or objective parameter?

Juhl
It is a subjective one; it is that minimal difference between the therapies that a physician would consider relevant to his decision of how a patient should be treated.

Tygstrup It can be specified in objective terms; for instance, it may be a 10% difference in the number of patients surviving 5 years.

Juhl
Clinical significance may be 10% for you, but perhaps it is 20% for me, and therefore in my opinion it is a subjective concept.

Riis
We usually consider the minimal relevant difference by asking ourselves: would a 2% difference be decisive for us?, would 8%?, or 10%? Of course this is not an exact method, but if several physicians are asked to state what would be clinically significant, they will cluster around a given figure.

Ingelfinger
Usually the problem is that we miss detecting a clinically relevant therapeutic effect due to a sample size too small, but sometimes we have a statistically significant effect of no clinical relevance. A good example is the influence of blood groups in the diagnosis of duodenal ulcer. Statistically, if one takes thousands of people, one might find say 52% of patients with ulcers to be in group O, and 48% in groups A or B, compared to the usual prevalence of 50% in group O in the normal population. This is statistically very significant with such a large sample size. But it is such a small difference that when a patient seeks therapy, it does not help very much in making a diagnosis. In this case,

the difference is highly significant statistically, but only minimally significant, if at all, clinically.

Active Controls versus Placebo Controls

Blum
A difficult problem for the clinicians in many studies is the choice of the control group. As an example, consider the study of acute pancreatitis. Let us assume that we plan to conduct a controlled trial to determine whether a lipid-reducing agent lowers the mortality of acute pancreatitis. Should this be compared with placebo or with another drug for which an effect in the treatment of acute pancreatitis has already been established? Several hundred trials on the treatment of acute pancreatitis have been published, but only a few of them were controlled, and only one trial by Trapnell et al. (2) claimed that a drug was effective. It was shown that a trypsin-inhibiting agent, Trasylol, significantly lowers the mortality of this disease (7% versus 25% with placebo). On first sight, it would appear that Trasylol is an effective treatment for pancreatitis. One might therefore conclude that in a new trial the lipid-reducing agent should be compared with Trasylol rather than a placebo.

The trial by Trapnell et al., however, has several shortcomings. First, placebo and Trasylol were given in ampules which were labeled as A or B. Such labeling is dangerous, since the trial is no longer double-blind if the code of any individual patient is broken during an emergency. Furthermore, the labeling of the drugs with A and B facilitates the development of prejudice for or against a certain treatment since only treatment group identity was blinded, not individual treatment assignment, i.e., all patients in group A were known to be in group A. Had the medication been continuously numbered, the treating physician would have been less likely to become prejudiced during the trial.

Second, the code was in fact broken when 49 patients had been treated, but since statistical significance was not reached, the trial was continued to the point when 105 patients had been treated. Dr. Chalmers (3) and others (4) have shown that the likelihood of reaching statistical significance rises each time a sample is examined and a statistical test conducted. After the second analysis a p-value which normally would indicate statistical significance might not be applicable anymore.

The Trasylol trial therefore illustrates that the double-blind and randomization do not protect a trial from being inconclusive. It depends as well on how the trial was conducted. In my opinion, Trasylol has not been proven to be an effective treatment of acute pancreatitis and a new drug would rather be compared with placebo than with Trasylol.

Repeated Significance Tests

Riis
Was it wrong to use significance levels when performing repeated significance tests at roughly 50 and 100 patients?

Lachin
On the second look at the data the sample size has been doubled, and it has been shown mathematically that the total probability of reaching a false positive conclusion has risen from 5 to 8% (4; see also section 9.5). So it happens every time another statistical test is conducted. Sooner or later, by making repeated statistical tests, the probability is almost certain that one will reject the null hypothesis even if it is true. This is a problem not only for repeated looks at the accumulating data but also for statistical tests of multiple variables or across various subgroups of the sample. This is a major statistical consideration of which all clinicians should be aware since these types of multiple analyses are often of greatest clinical interest.

REFERENCES

1. Lachin, J. M., Marks, J. W., Schoenfield, L. J., and the NCGS Protocol Committee, and the National Cooperative Gallstone Study Group, Design and methodological considerations in the National Cooperative Gallstone Study: A multicenter clinical trial. Controlled Clinical Trials, 1981, 2, 177-230.
2. Trapnell, J. E., Rigby, C. C., Talboth, C. H., and Duncan, H. L., A controlled trial of trasylol in the treatment of acute pancreatitis. Br. J. Surg., 1974, 61, 177-182.
3. Chalmers, T. C., Randomize the first patient. N. Engl. J. Med., 1977, 296, 107.
4. McPherson, K., Statistics: The problem of examining accumulating data more than once. N. Engl. J. Med., 1975, 290, 501-502.

ADDITIONAL READINGS

Feinstein, A., Clinical Biostatistics, C. V. Mosby, St. Louis, Mo., 1977.

Tygstrup, N., and Juhl, E., Dilemmas of controlled clinical trials in hepatology, in The Liver and Its Diseases (F. Schaffner, S. Sherlock, and C. M. Leevy, eds.), Intercontinental Medical Book Corporation, New York, 1974, pp. 64-75.

5
Principles for Selection and Exclusion

ANDRÉ L. BLUM
Triemli Hospital
Zurich, Switzerland

The basic objective of a clinical trial is to describe the effects of a therapy in comparison to what would be observed if the standard, or no therapy, were applied to a population of ill patients. The patient population to which the results apply is defined according to the criteria for patient selection and exclusion, the principles for which are explored in this chapter.

Throughout this chapter it is important to distinguish between the actual sample, or group of patients actually studied, and the population to which the results are to be applied. The population refers to the usually infinite class of all individual patients which might have been selected for randomization into the study, while the sample refers to the finite number of patients actually randomized into the study.

5.1 A LABORATORY EXPERIMENT

As an analogy, consider an animal experiment using a sample of four mice randomized into two groups of two mice each. Except for the small number of participants, which has been chosen for the sake of simplicity, this represents an ideal situation. Laboratory mice closely resemble each other, the population from which the sample is drawn is homogeneous, and the two study groups can easily be compared. Circumstances like these, however, are rarely encountered in randomized, controlled trials.

Now assume that we are not satisfied by performing a trial in mice only and that we decide to admit any four legged mammal to the study. As it turns out, by chance two mice and two elephants enter the trial and randomization assigns one mouse and one elephant to each group. The two study groups are again quite similar, but they lack homogeneity. Assume that we treat one group with placebo and the other with a medication which is effective in 100% of those properly treated. It is clearly evident that a dose which is sufficient to treat a mouse is far below the dose which would affect an elephant. Conversely, a dose which is necessary to treat an elephant will kill a mouse. In such a heterogeneous sample, therefore, the proportion of successes in the treated group is likely not to be 100%, but rather 50% at best, and under certain circumstances we will even get the impression that the active medication has failed.

In this mouse and elephant study, there is an additional distressing possibility. So far we have assumed that randomization in a heterogeneous population would lead to a similar composition of the two groups. This is not necessarily so, and randomization could have assigned two elephants to one group and two mice to the other, thus leading to misleading results. If somehow we were not aware of this fact, the results of the study would lead to an erroneous conclusion. Lack of homogeneity of the population studied in a trial, therefore, is always disturbing, because it could lead to an imbalance in the composition of the groups.

One way to deal with this problem is to specify an appropriate subpopulation within the larger nonhomogeneous population from which the study sample will be drawn. In our animal study we might have selected only those animals which belong to one of the common laboratory species, thus excluding inappropriate classes of subjects such as elephants. The population to be studied is now more homogeneous, and a sample of subjects can be randomized without any difficulty.

Principles for Selection and Exclusion 45

This advantage, however, is offset by two difficulties. First, due to the selection criteria, the population that can be sampled to obtain subjects is only half as large as it was originally. Second, and perhaps even worse, the trial only deals with laboratory species and not with elephants, and therefore is only of very limited value if we really wanted information about the treatment of four-legged mammals in general.

Another possibility for dealing with heterogeneity exists when a method is available to reliably differentiate the study subjects on prognostic criteria, that is, mice from elephants. In this case, the next logical step is prerandomization prognostic stratification (Figure 5.1). By this process mice are separated from elephants and the two types of

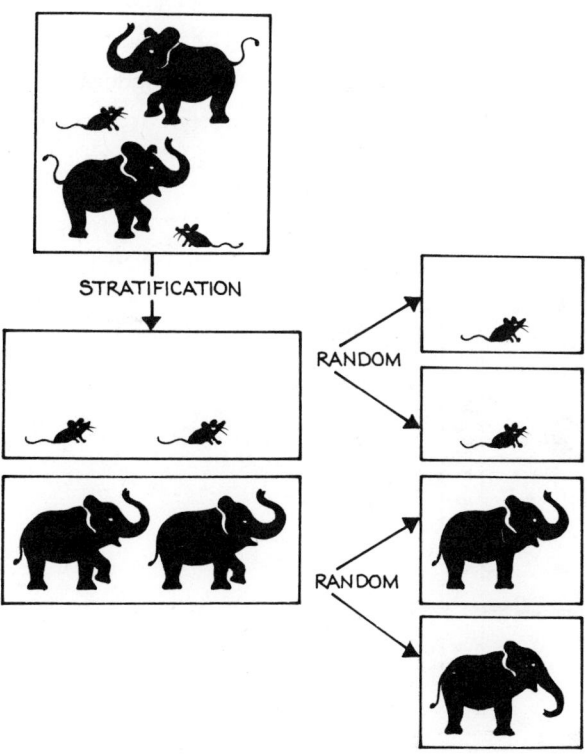

FIGURE 5.1 Prognostic prerandomization stratification.

46 Blum

animals are randomized and then analyzed separately. Thus, no type of animal is lost to the study.

5.2 THE CLINICAL TRIAL

Now switch from animals to humans. Since we differ in many respects from mice, a homogeneous population is only obtained through the specification of criteria for the selection of the patients to enter the trial.

Responders and Nonresponders

Assume we are planning to conduct a trial in a disease with a broad spectrum of severity (Figure 5.2). It may affect the patient with only minor symptoms, or it may appear as a disease of moderate severity, or it may be a very serious disease with a poor prognosis. Without treatment the seriously ill patient will soon die. The almost healthy individual, however, may recover spontaneously, and the moderately ill patient may remain unchanged. Assume that an active treatment is

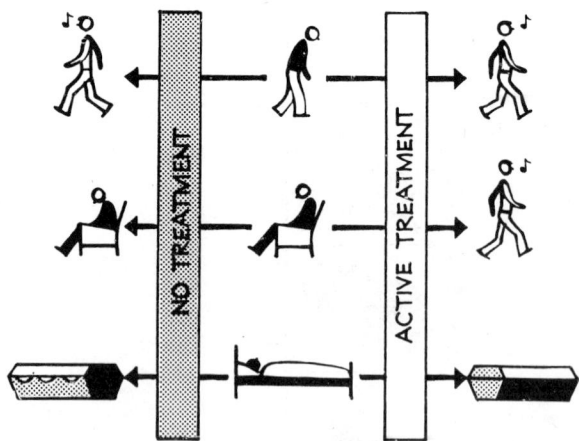

FIGURE 5.2 Severity of illness and improvement with or without treatment.

Principles for Selection and Exclusion 47

now applied to these patients. The moderately ill patient and the almost healthy patient both recover, while the seriously ill patient dies. Thus, a response to treatment can only be observed in the moderately ill patient, while the two extremes, the almost healthy and the seriously ill, are nonresponders for two different reasons: spontaneous recovery or inevitable death.

In a broader sense any disease population consists of good responders and bad responders and usually also an intermediate group which may either respond or not respond to treatment. Thus, unless selection criteria are adopted, it is inevitable that the population studied will be heterogeneous and will yield subgroups with different prognoses and different responses to treatment.

As an example, consider the effects of selection criteria in three different hypothetical studies of the prophylactic effects of carbenoxolene in the treatment of duodenal ulcer (Table 5.1). In study A, imaginary hospitalized patients without prior ulcer attacks, having newly diagnosed, endoscopically proven ulcers, are studied. In these patients the prognosis is very good, with or without carbenoxolene, since the ulcers are likely to have been small and of short duration, and because hospitalization would also include reduced smoking and alcohol intake. In study B, outpatients with newly diagnosed, endoscopically proven ulcers are studied. It is not specified whether they may have had prior attacks, but the overall prognosis is expected to be neither excellent nor poor. Study C employs outpatients with chronic recurrent, radiologically proven ulcers. For these patients the prognosis is very poor, and there is no reason to expect a tendency to respond to carbenoxolene.

As could be expected, these three studies lead to different conclusions. In study A, 83% healed when treated only with placebo. Carbenoxolone did not significantly improve this near-maximal healing rate. In study C the proportion healed with placebo is poor. Healing tends to be somewhat more rapid with carbenoxolone, but among the 60

TABLE 5.1 Effects of Prognosis on Outcome in Three Hypothetical Ulcer Trials

	Study A (1)	Study B (2)	Study C (3)
Previous ulcer attacks	None	2	>2
Duration of present attack	<1 month	<1 month	<2 months
Diagnosis	Endoscopy	Endoscopy	Radiology
Small ulcers likely to be included	Yes	Yes	No
Hospitalization	Yes	No	No
Likely to give up drinking	Yes	No	No
Likely to give up smoking	?	No	No
Healed within 6 weeks			
Placebo	83%	48%	12%
Carbenoxolone	89%	75%	18%
Difference	n.s.	$p < 0.01$	n.s.
Sample size (N)	60	60	60

patients studied the difference is not statistically significant. In study B, the proportion healed with placebo is 48% and with carbenoxolone it is 75%. This difference is statistically significant.

These three studies demonstrate that the patient selection criteria markedly affect the outcome of a trial. An effect may or may not be observed, depending on how the patient population to be studied is defined.

5.3 PROGNOSTIC STRATIFICATION

The randomized clinical trial is an attempt to introduce the scientific method into everyday clinical medicine. Diagnostic selection criteria in clinical trials, however, are usually more restrictive than those encountered in everyday medicine. A diagnosis which under ordinary circumstances is quite acceptable might not be acceptable in a clinical trial. On the other hand, if the diagnostic criteria of a clinical trial are too far removed from everyday medicine, the results of the trial may not be applicable to clinical practice. This would be a serious drawback because the main purpose of a trial is, after all, to improve the everyday practice of medicine and not just to obtain significant results among homogeneous populations. One approach to this dilemma is to employ heterogeneous diagnostic selection criteria and then evaluate the various diagnostic subgroups separately in the final statistical analyses.

As an example, consider that we wish to evaluate whether an acid secretion blocking agent is effective in promoting the healing of gastric ulcers. There are three types of gastric ulcers. Type I is located in the gastric body, type III is located near the pylorus, and type II is combined with the duodenal ulcer. Acid plays a major role in the pathogenesis of type II, a small role in type III, and a negligible role in type I. On the other hand, drugs, alcohol, and nicotine play a major role in the pathogenesis of type I, a smaller role in type III, and a negligible role in type II gastric ulcers.

It should be expected, therefore, that antisecretory agents are likely to be effective in type II ulcers, less likely to be effective in type III ulcers, and least likely to be effective in type I ulcers. Assume that this indeed is the case. Among all three types of ulcers, approximately 40% heal spontaneously (e.g., on placebo) within 12 weeks. When treated with antisecretory agents, the proportion healed among type II ulcers increases to almost 75%, the healing rate of type I ulcers is not affected, and type III ulcers display an intermediate response. Since the type of ulcer is readily diagnosable, it is clear that ulcer type will likely be a highly prognostic indicator of success with antisecretory drug therapy.

Table 5.2 presents the results which might have been obtained from two hypothetical separate studies conducted in each of two countries (A and B) with differing prevalences of the three ulcer types. In each study 200 patients with any of the three ulcer types were randomized without consideration of ulcer type, i.e., using a simple randomization plan without stratification. Thus, the numbers randomized into each treatment group in each country reflect approximately the prevalence of that ulcer type within that country.

In country A, type I and III ulcers predominate almost equally (45% prevalence), and the total proportion healed in the drug-treated group is 53% as compared to 40% in the placebo group. The statistical test of the difference between the two groups is not significant. Thus, although the drug does in truth affect certain types of gastric ulcers, notably type II, this effect is not demonstrated by the total healing rates. Therefore, due to lack of homogeneity in the population, the study showed a small overall therapeutic effect (53% versus 40% healed), but with an insufficient sample size to account for this heterogeneity, an effect which was actually present was not demonstrated statistically. In this case a total sample size of 506 would have been required to yield 90% probability (power) of reaching a significant difference in overall healing rates, ($\alpha = 0.05$, one-sided).

Note, however, that among type II ulcers the proportion healed in the drug group was 75% compared to 44% with placebo, but again due to small sample size, statistical significance was not achieved, 86 type II patients being necessary to yield 90% power of reaching significance.

In country B, however, type II ulcers predominate, 138 patients with type II ulcers having entered the study. This sample size provides 90% power of reaching statistical significance. As a result a highly

TABLE 5.2 Hypothetical Trials of an Antisecretory Agent in Treatment of Gastric Ulcer, Performed in Two Countries with Different Prevalence Rates of the Three Main Ulcer Types, 200 Patients in Each Trial

		% Healed	
Ulcer type	% Prevalence	Drug	Placebo
Country A			
I (drug dependent)	45.0	38.1 (16/42)	42.5 (20/47)
II (acid dependent)	10.0	75.0 (9/12)	44.4 (4/9)
III (intermediate)	45.0	60.9 (28/46)	36.4 (16/44)
Total	100.0	53.0 (53/100)	40.0 (40/100)
$\chi^2 = 2.89$ $p = 0.09$ (n.s.)			
Country B			
I (drug dependent)	15.0	35.3 (6/17)	42.9 (6/14)
II (acid dependent)	70.0	69.1 (47/68)	38.6 (27/70)
III (intermediate)	15.0	46.7 (7/15)	43.8 (7/16)
Total	100.0	60.0 (60/100)	40.0 (40/100)
$\chi^2 = 7.22$ $p < 0.01$			

statistically significant therapeutic effect is observed among type II ulcers ($\chi^2 = 11.74$, $p < 0.001$), and also among all ulcer types combined.

From these observations it is apparent that when there is prognostic heterogeneity, a false negative (β) error may be committed if prognostic stratification is not accounted for in the planning and the statistical analysis. If, on the other hand, the population studied is prognostically homogeneous, stratification is not useful, and further the selection criteria might in themselves lead to an increased type II error by restricting the potential sample size of the study.

5.4 COMPLIANCE

Finally, there is the very difficult problem of the compliance of the patient with the treatment, which will be discussed in the next chapter. In this context, however, it should be emphasized that the expected compliance with treatment might closely be associated with other patient characteristics. For example, assume that the ulcer patients with good compliance do not tend to excessive intake of alcohol, nicotine, or drugs. In this group of patients, type II and type III ulcers are relatively frequent. In contrast, patients whose estimated compliance is poor may have predominantly type I ulcers. If a trial is conducted only among compliant patients, there would likely be a significant difference between treatment and placebo because few patients with type I ulcers would be included. This example demonstrates that compliance to treatment is often associated with important characteristics of the disease and should also be considered in planning the selection criteria for a clinical trial.

5.5 DISCUSSION

Patient Selection versus Generalization of Results

Schoenfield

Dr. Blum has described the importance of selection criteria, but there are additional considerations in choosing selection criteria. First, specific types of patients should be excluded if inclusion in the study would thereby place these patients at some increased risk to their well-being or health. Second, and perhaps in conflict with the first consideration, the patient population studied should be relevant to the population for whom the therapy will ultimately be used. Criteria for selection that are too rigid should not be employed because the study will not apply to the general population and the results will not be of general clinical use. Thus, we have the dilemma of using loose criteria in which patients are characterized by many variables or using rigid criteria in which there may be a loss of generality.

Ingelfinger
I wonder if broad generalizations on the basis of a randomized trial are ever feasible. The more we restrict the eligible population's characteristics (one age group, one sex, one blood-pressure level, and so on), the more accurate and valid we probably make the study, but we also restrict the possibility of generalizing its results to the larger population. As far as I can see, the more accurate the randomized trial, the less its results can be generalized to the population at large.

Riis
The choice of selection criteria can have a tremendous influence on the results. One trial may study seriously ill nonresponders, while another trial may study good responders, and the results will be very different. The problem, however, is that the trial producing negative results due to the selection of nonresponders is usually not reported.

Juhl
We conducted a multicenter trial comparing prednisone with placebo in cirrhosis (1). Among patients randomized into the trial, the survival curves for the prednisone and placebo groups were not significantly different. In spite of broad admission criteria, however, only 30% of the patients screened were included in the trial, but all patients were followed. The survival curves of the patients who entered the trial and those who were excluded are significantly different, with a slightly better prognosis for patients included and assigned to receive placebo (Figure 5.3). This result shows how important the criteria for selection and exclusion really are.

Chalmers
Figure 5.4 presents the similar results of a study of portacaval shunt surgery conducted in Boston (2). We have added the survival curve for those rejected from the study, generally because they were considered high surgical risks. Clearly, the best survival is among those selected for the trial (i.e,. selected for surgery) but who were assigned to the nonsurgical control group.

One of the problems with this study, however, is that this was a study predominantly of poorer, public assistance patients. In the United States, the wealthier patients pay for their own medical care, and their physicians often feel that since they are being paid to care for their patients and to make decisions, that it is not right for their private patients to be randomized into a study. In the United States, perhaps 90% of randomized patients are not private patients. Thus, in many countries there is an automatic selection bias in that only poor people are randomized, and based on socioeconomic related factors, the poor

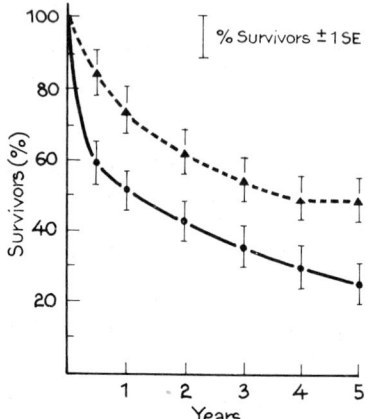

FIGURE 5.3 Percentage of survivors ±SE by year after randomization for those admitted to the clinical trial (▲) and those excluded from admission (●). (From Ref. 1.)

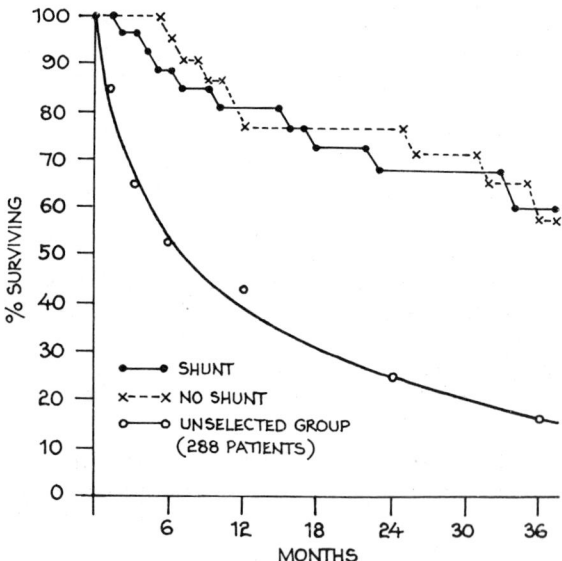

FIGURE 5.4 Survival from onset of varices of the study groups compared with survival of 288 unselected patients with varices without hemorrhage. (From Ref. 2. Reprinted, by permission of the N. Engl. J. Med., 1964, 270, 496-500.)

may or may not be good responders to therapy. The unfortunate thing about the Boston study is that we still do not know about the efficacy of portacaval shunt surgery in private patients.

Schoenfield
I think it is a misconception, however, that private patients will not be willing to participate in a randomized trial. I believe that if the patients are approached properly, if it is explained to them why the study is being conducted and how carefully the trial was developed, then this will not hold true. I have been involved in three clinical trials in which we had no difficulties recruiting private patients. The patients do not object; only their doctors think they will.

Stratification

Wright
There are many clinical situations in which stratification is very relevant. For instance, there may be a great difference in the response to corticosteroids in patients with ulcerative colitis during their first attack as opposed to chronic cases. I would like to ask the statisticians whether prospective stratification is so much more valuable than retrospective stratification in the analysis of one's data.

Lachin
I generally do not advocate prospective, prerandomization stratification for a number of reasons, one of which is that many methods of statistical analysis can be employed to do two things. First, any imbalance between the treatment groups on a prognostic variable can be accounted for in the analysis. For example, when there are more females in group A than in group B, and thus more patients in group A among females, the analysis can actually adjust for this imbalance. Second, these same methods can also account for different event rates within subgroups. For example, in the gastric ulcer study, the data could be analyzed accounting for the different treatment effects seen in the ulcer type subgroups. Both these features are illustrated in Chapter 11. Overall, therefore, I feel that the methods of analysis are so generally applicable and powerful that there is little utility to prerandomization stratification, especially with its difficulties in implementation.

Tygstrup
I think that we are dealing with two problems. One is to randomize several strata separately in order to ensure equal representation of each stratum in the treatment and control groups, i.e., to reduce the risk of "bad luck randomization." The other problem is to stratify in order to see if different types of patients with the target disease react differently to the treatment. In the first case only one comparison is made between treated patients and controls; whereas in the second case each stratum is analyzed separately. In other words, the trial is broken

down into a number of smaller trials with the risk of greater type II error.

Lachin
Actually, with or without prerandomization stratification the data can be analyzed separately within each strata, and in both cases, pooled analyses should also be conducted across strata. The pooled overall comparison of treatment versus control then will have greater power, i.e., less type II error, than the individual subgroup comparisons. Thus, the main use of stratification should be to evaluate subgroup effects in the analysis, and for this prospective stratification is usually not necessary. Further, stratified randomization to ensure balanced subgroups is usually not necessary since simple randomization with a large sample size yields a very small probability that a severe imbalance will occur.

Checking Randomization

Riis
Published reports of randomized trials state the sex ratio, age, and a lot of other variables for each treatment group, and sometimes statistical tests are presented for each variable. Isn't this unnecessary, since the risk of having an imbalance on a concomitant factor is included in the type I error level of the statistical test?

Tygstrup
Is it reasonable to test the randomization by comparing the groups with respect to other variables of interest?

Lachin
Even though randomization is used to induce comparability, there is always the possibility that an imbalance on one or more important variables might occur. Even though the final statistical test could be conducted with a specified type I error level α without having looked for the effects of imbalances, I think the investigator should always explore this possibility and evaluate the success of the randomization.

Tygstrup
How is this done, by a separate test on each measured variable? For example, did males fare better than females?

Lachin
First we look (or if you wish, test) to see whether there is an imbalance on each prognostic variable among the groups (e.g., more females in the treated group than control). If so, the data are further examined to see if there is a differential treatment effect, e.g., do females respond differently from males. In doing so, however, we have to realize that due to the multiplicity of tests, by chance some comparisons will be significant. Suppose one uses the α level 0.05. If we have 100 variables

to be evaluated, the probability may be as high as 0.995 that 1 or more of the 100 variables will be significant by chance alone. Even for only 10 variables, this overall type I error may be as high as 0.40 (3). The exact overall α level is difficult to evaluate since it depends on the number of variables tested and the correlations between them. The main point, however, is that the investigator should examine the differences between the groups, and if the groups are shown to be imbalanced, this should be accounted for in the analysis. It is important that we not assume that because we randomized we are not going to get an imbalance.

Tygstrup
We also have the problem that a highly prognostic variable was simply unknown and was not even recorded, and it may have an imbalance between the groups.

Lachin
That, of course, is why it is very difficult to be sure of anything. There are no simple answers to these types of problems. The best recommendation is to be extremely thorough in planning, executing, and analyzing a study. All avenues should be explored even if they raise more questions than answers.

REFERENCES

1. Juhl, E., Holden, M., and Tygstrup, N., Effect of selection in controlled clinical trials. Scand. J. Gastroent., 1971, 9, 171-175.

2. Garceau, A. J., Donaldson, R. M., O'Hara, E. T., Callow, A. D., Muench, H., Chalmers, T. C., and the Boston Inter-Hospital Liver Group, A controlled trial of prophylactic portacaval-shunt surgery. N. Engl. J. Med., 1964, 270, 496-500.

3. Kupper, L. L., Steward, J. R. and Williams, K. A., A note on controlling significance levels in stepwise regression. Amer. J. Epidemiol., 1976, 103, 13-15.

6
Clinical Evaluation of Success

ANDRÉ L. BLUM
Triemli Hospital
Zurich, Switzerland

The ideal form of a clinical trial is like the 100-m dash at a track meet. The trial starts for all participants at the same moment, and the evaluation of success is simple and straightforward. Only one value plays a role, the time from the start to the finish line, and this can be exactly measured by a watch. Most importantly, the measured performance of the participants is independent of the observer.

This is quite different in clinical trials. Evaluation of success in most instances is not independent of the observer, and therefore, this evaluation is a difficult task. There have been cases in which the observer's bias is stronger than his feelings for scientific objectivity, and after starting the trial, he changes the rules. This is an obvious and frequent mistake in clinical trials. Therefore, a very rigid and clearcut protocol should be followed for the evaluation of the effects of therapy.

6.1 MULTIPLE FACTORS

In clinical trials, evaluation of success is complicated in either or both of two ways. First, individuals entering a trial usually can be characterized by many variables or factors, and these many factors may affect the outcome of treatment. In this case, many different types of

TABLE 6.1 Criteria for Evaluation of Treatment Success Using Peptic Ulcer as an Example

Criterion	Subjective measures	Objective measures
Course of disease	Mild pain only?	No radiologic evidence of ulcer growth
Complications of disease	Any vomiting, blood in stool?	Blood hematocrit levels
Healing rate	Soon pain free?	Endoscopically proven ulcer healing
Relapse rate	Any dyspepsia after healing?	Endoscopically proven ulcer healing
Side effects	Any headaches?	Hypertension demonstrated by systolic blood pressure >110 mmHg
Treatment convenience	Missed taking medication?	Percentage adherence (capsules taken versus those prescribed)
Mortality		Time to death, cause of death

statistical analyses can be performed to parcel out the importance of these various prognostic factors.

Second, and much more problematic, is the fact that the outcome of a trial is usually evaluated by more than just one measurement. The treatment may affect the course of the disease or the frequency of relapses, it may have side affects, and it may cost less than previous treatments. Here the investigator can either examine single outcomes individually, or give a general impression about the multiple outcomes of the trial, or use composite indices for the outcome evaluation, such as those derived as linear combinations in multivariate analysis.

Unfortunately, in most clinical trials the participants are characterized by many factors at the beginning of the trial and many effects are observed at the end. Under these circumstances evaluation is very difficult, and a simple recipe cannot be given.

In most clinical trials seven basic criteria can be used for the evaluation of success (Table 6.1), either with subjective or objective outcome measures. For example, in a trial of gastric ulcers the course may be less severe when an active medication is given, the patient complains only of mild pain, and the ulcer does not grow during the treatment period. In addition, there are also subjective and objective measures of the grade of complications, healing rate, relapses, side effects, and the convenience of treatment.

It is well known that very serious statistical problems arise when more than one variable is evaluated. In fact, when seven variables are evaluated separately, there may be as high as 30% probability that at least one significant result at the 0.05 level will occur by chance. Seven variables are not too many, and therefore, we are heading for trouble.

6.2 CLINICAL IMPRESSIONS

One way to avoid some of these difficulties is to use an overall general impression or judgment about the effects of treatment. Such subjective evaluations, however, are not without pitfalls. As an example, Figure 6.1 shows the results of a double-blind study conducted to evaluate premedication with diazepam versus placebo for endoscopy (1) where the endoscopists rated premedication as successful or not successful according to how cooperatively the patient behaved during the examination. The results are reported as the percentage of successful premedications in successive groups of 50 patients. Throughout the

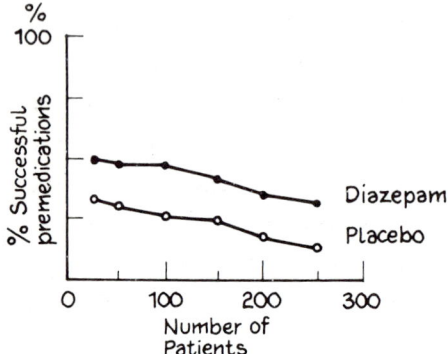

FIGURE 6.1 Endoscopist's judgment. Cumulative percentage of success with diazepam and placebo assessed by the endoscopist as each group of 50 patients were examined. (Data from Ref. 1.)

entire study diazepam was better than placebo, but the endoscopist inadvertently became more and more critical in his judgment. Among the first 50 patients 50% of the placebo-treated and 70% of the diazepam-treated patients were rated as successful premedication. Among the last 50 patients the success rates were 30 and 50%, respectively. Thus, the success rate of diazepam at the end of the study was similar to the success rate of placebo at the beginning.

This change in success rates could be due to a change in the attitude or standard of evaluation of the endoscopist or to an improvement in the experience and skill of the endoscopist thus affecting patient behavior, although in the latter case a decline in the percentage of success would not be expected. In any event, this example clearly shows that general impressions are subject to change in the course of a study. Inadvertently the observer may acquire a more critical or a less critical attitude.

6.3 DIRECT VERSUS INDIRECT MEASURES OF THERAPEUTIC EFFECTS

Chapter 5 discussed a hypothetical trial in gastric ulcer (Table 5.2), in which the therapy was evaluated using the rate of ulcers healed.

Healing of a gastric ulcer, however, is difficult to evaluate because the time taken to heal varies and because an invasive procedure (radiology or endoscopy) is required to determine healing. It might be argued, therefore, that instead of healing, it would be better to use a parameter easier to quantify, such as gastric secretion.

Referring to Table 5.2, healing rate with an antisecretory agent is highly dependent on ulcer type, and in country A, due to a low prevalence of acid-induced type II ulcers, the overall healing rates were not significantly different: 53% on treatment versus 40% on placebo. Gastric secretion levels, however, are not influenced by ulcer type. If the criteria for success were a 50% reduction in basal acid output levels, the trial would likely display 0% successes among the 100 placebo-treated patients and 90% successes among those on the drug, both overall and among each ulcer type, a highly statistically significant effect.

In the placebo group, however, 40% of the ulcers healed even though acid secretion was not reduced. In the drug group, reduction of secretion would likely be similar among patients who healed and those who did not. From these results it would be apparent that the degree to which gastric secretion is reduced is not directly related to clinical success.

In general, distinction can be made between _direct_ and _indirect_ _measures_ of therapeutic effects. An easily quantified indirect effect (secretion) may not be related to a direct evaluation of therapeutic effect (healing). Thus, if we want to know whether a drug promotes healing of gastric ulcer, healing should be the outcome measure rather than the more easily quantified rate of gastric secretions, because the two in this case are likely not to be related.

6.4. CLINICAL SCORES

We have already heard it is difficult to evaluate a multiplicity of outcomes in a controlled study. For example, in the studies of gastric ulcer, we may want to know whether a drug also improves ulcer symptoms, such as the frequency of attacks of pain, the intensity of pain, the duration of the attacks, or additional symptoms such as nausea and the number of antacid tablets taken.

In such cases we may decide to use a clinical score to evalute the success of treatment. In Table 6.2 is an example how such a score might be constructed. The patient gets one point when he or she has had one attack of pain per day and two points with two or more attacks a day; one point when the intensity of the pain was light, and so on. Thus, a patient's total score can range between 0 and 10 points.

Some feel that composite clinical scores are the answer to all the difficulties in clinical evaluation since they replace subjective impressions by numerical values. More than one effect can be evaluated in a study, and it provides a readily understood description of therapeutic effects, e.g., the patient has just improved from +8 to +2 points. I personally feel that clinical scores give a false impression of security to the attending physician. The thinking process which leads to

TABLE 6.2 A Clinical Score for Evaluation of Severity of Ulcer Symptoms

Symptom	Score	(Points)
Frequency of attacks	1/day =	1
	2/day =	2
Intensity of pain	Light =	1
	Strong =	2
Duration of attacks	<1 hr =	1
	>1 hr =	2
Additional symptoms	Yes =	2
Number of antacids	1-3 =	1
	>3 =	2
Total		0 to 10

a clinical impression is the same as that leading to a clinical score. The biased mind which would give a biased clinical impression about improvement would also allocate a biased number to the clinical score.

I even think that a clinician's judgment might be better than his score values. Imagine that a patient comes back after treatment and says, "Oh doctor, I feel much better." His physician actually has the same impression, but after calculating his score says, "No, Sir. You're worse!" How can this happen? Suppose that before treatment the frequency of attacks was four per day and during treatment, two per day, the intensity of pain decreased from very strong to strong, the duration of pain from 2 to 1 hr, and the nausea remained unchanged. However, a friend of the patient felt that the patient's physician had prescribed a medication which was actually too strong and he suggested that the patient take antacids which the patient had not taken before. In order not to disappoint his physician and his friend, the patient took both medications. This supercompliance scores one point. The score has risen from 8 to 9. Such examples show that composite clinical scores are by no means better than good clinical judgment.

6.5 STRATIFICATION

I would like to reemphasize the importance of stratification in the evaluation of treatment outcome. It was mentioned in Chapter 5 that a false negative result might be obtained without consideration of stratification when the difference between the prognostic groups is large. A few years ago a controlled study of estrogen treatment for advanced prostatic cancer (2) was performed (Table 6.3). Overall it appears that estrogen is not beneficial in prostatic cancer, death rates being between 16 and 20% in all groups.

Let us now stratify on the severity of the disease. Stage III prostatic cancer shows invasion into the pelvic tissue but no bone metastases. In stage IV there are bone metastases or metastases into other organs. Without estrogen treatment mortality is about 10% (7 of

TABLE 6.3 Trial of Multiple Doses of Estrogen in Treatment of Prostatic Cancer

	Dose of estrogen (mg/day)			
	0	0.2	1.0	5.0
Overall				
Death rate, %	18.8 (24/128)	20.0 (25/125)	16.4 (21/128)	19.7 (25/127)
Cause of death				
Cancer	10	12	4	4
Other	14	13	17	21
Stage III				
Death rate, %	9.3 (7/75)	15 (11/73)	19.2 (14/73)	21.9^a (16/73)
Cause of death				
Cancer	2	0	1	1
Other	5	11	13	15
Stage IV				
Death rate, %	32.0 (17/53)	26.9 (14/52)	12.7^a (7/55)	16.7 (9/54)
Cause of death				
Cancer	8	12	3	3
Other	9	2	4	6

$^a p < 0.05$ for chi-square test compared to zero dose.
Source: Data from Ref. 2.

75) in stage III and 33% in stage IV. In stage III, estrogen treatment clearly increases mortality due to an increased incidence of deaths from other causes, mostly cardiovascular, which represents an unwanted side effect. In stage IV, however, the higher doses of estrogen lowered the mortality because they reduced the incidence of cancer deaths. Again

Clinical Evaluation of Success   67

the same unwanted effect on cardiovascular disease is seen, but this is less marked because the patient with stage IV disease has a shorter life expectancy. Therefore, we may conclude that patients with stage III prostatic cancer should not be treated with estrogens, while patients with stage IV prostatic cancer should in fact receive such treatment. This study is a good example of the role of stratified or subgroup analyses and the delicate balance between wanted and unwanted effects of treatment.

6.6 PREMATURE EXITS FROM STUDY

Side effects of treatment may also seriously complicate a controlled study if they lead to a premature discontinuation of treatment or exit from the study by one or more patients. Assume that placebo is to be compared with a medication which has side effects but no benefical effect on the disease (Figure 6.2). Two patients are randomized to receive placebo: a patient who has only mild disease and recovers

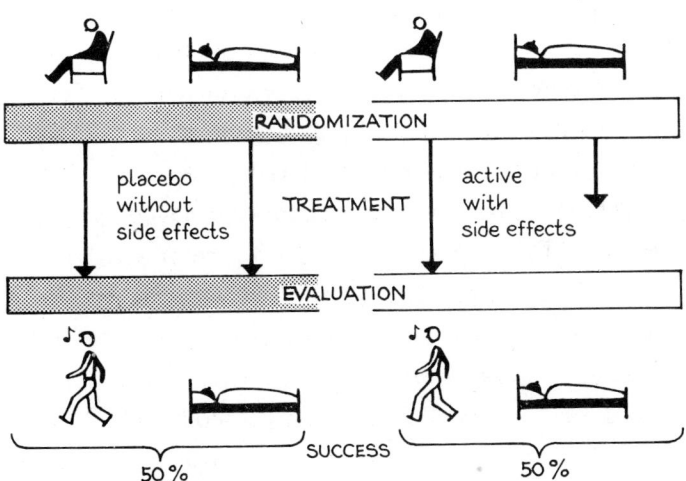

FIGURE 6.2 Premature withdrawals among those receiving placebo and active treatment.

spontaneously during placebo treatment and a seriously ill patient who remains seriously ill. Two patients are likewise allocated to receive the drug treatment. One is again a moderately ill patient who progresses to healing, although in the course of treatment he shows the side effects of the drug. The other, a seriously ill patient, shows the same side effects, and the combination of serious disease and side effects is so dangerous that the physician decides to stop treatment. After completion of the trial, the success rate is then evaluated, and it is 50% in both the placebo and the treatment group.

If we argue, however, that the patient in whom treatment was discontinued because of side effects does not belong in the analysis because he did not complete the entire course of active treatment, the success rate would clearly be 100%. In this case the active medication would appear to be twice as effective as placebo. We also know, however, that the active medication has no beneficial effect and that it is actually harmful due to its side effects. This example demonstrates that patients in whom treatment is discontinued because of side effects must remain in the group into which they were randomized. Removal of a patient from an assigned group may cause very serious bias.

Very often patients are excluded from analysis because, as the author claims, they have been lost to follow-up or dropped out. Such an exclusion might only be discussed when there is absolute certainty that the loss of the patient was completely unrelated to the study. This, however, is very rarely the case. When a patient has moved away, this may have been supported by an improvement due to treatment, or when a patient drops out, he may have been dissatisfied with the treatment and, therefore, saw another physician. Also, a patient may have died because of a side effect of the treatment, even a mild one. Patients have been known to die in automobile accidents caused by drug-induced dizziness. For these reasons, it is advisable not to exclude any patient from the study analysis once randomized.

Clinical Evaluation of Success   69

6.7 COMPLIANCE

Another serious problem is the compliance of the patient with treatment. In Figure 6.3 two compliant and two alcoholic patients who tend to be noncompliant are enrolled in a controlled study in which the treatment is actually effective in those properly treated. The compliant patient who gets the active treatment is healed, and the compliant patient who gets placebo treatment deteriorates. The two alcoholics do not improve. They discontinue treatment after a short while and they both deteriorate. In the placebo group the success rate is 0% among compliant patients, noncompliant patients, and overall. With active medication the success rate is 100% in the compliant patients. When the noncompliant patient is included, the success rate is only 50%. Therefore, the noncompliant patient gives a wrong

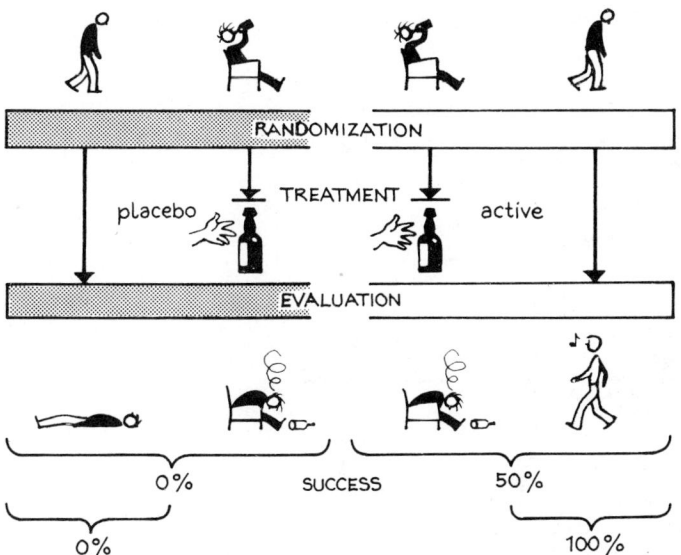

FIGURE 6.3 Compliance among those receiving placebo and active treatment.

70   Blum

impression of the drug's true efficacy. The drug is much more effective than is shown by the study. Should the noncompliant patients be removed from the analysis? I think not. Let me show you why.

Again, two alcoholic and two nonalcoholic patients are treated (Figure 6.4). Again, the drug has a beneficial effect, but the disease has a tendency for spontaneous healing. Assume that the compliant patients in each group heal spontaneously. The treated alcoholic patient is improved by the therapy, and therefore complies with therapy despite the alcoholism. The other alcoholic patient who gets placebo treatment is not improved, becomes noncompliant, increases alcohol intake, and deteriorates.

In this case there is a close relationship between the effect of treatment and the compliance with treatment. If the patient who discontinued treatment was excluded, the success rate in the placebo group would be 100%, the same as for the patients on active medication. If the noncompliant patient is retained, however, the

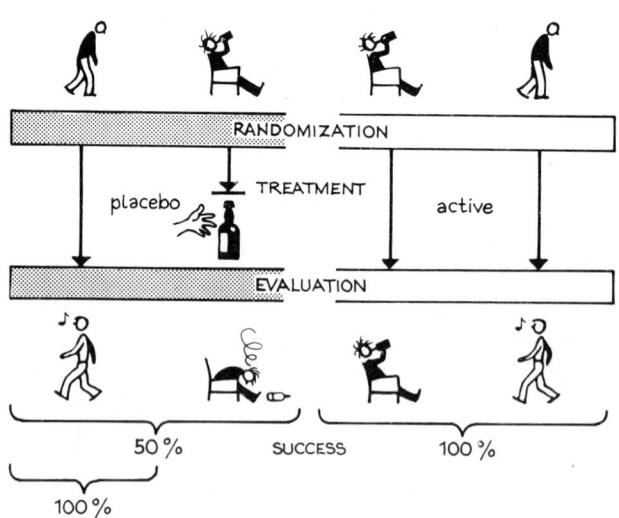

FIGURE 6.4 Compliance interacting with treatment.

beneficial effect of the treatment is apparent. The success rate in the placebo group is now 50%, and in the group with active medication it is 100%.

In order to avoid problems with compliance, many investigations perform so-called trial periods during which all patients receive placebo medication. Randomization is only performed with whose patients who comply during this period. In the above example, the two alcoholic noncompliant patients would hopefully drop out during the trial period and would not be randomized. Hopefully only compliant patients are then randomized. This again leads, however, to the problem of selection. The results of the trial can only then be applied to compliant patients with uncomplicated disease, noncompliant patients with serious disease not having been studied. And the effects of treatment in these latter patients would not be known.

6.8 DISCUSSION

Clinical Scores

Chalmers
I take objection to the statement that clinical scores are bad. If scores are expressed with sound judgment, I would be more confident in them than a physician's general impression. An outstanding example is the study of Crohn's disease (3), a symptom complex of wide range and severity with no direct measure of "healing." We thus adopted a clinical score which was used with great success (4).

Ingelfinger
I want to pursue the same objection. You have proposed that a clinical trial be undertaken according to elaborate statistical guidelines, and then the result evaluated by a totally invalid criterion, namely clinical judgment. One day we may feel very upset; the stock market is going down, so we mark everything poor. Another day we feel very happy; we are going to Italy, so we mark everything up. It is true that by randomization and blinding the comparison possibly will not be greatly affected, but I don't think one can get a true overall picture unless there are precise evaluation criteria. It seems to me this destroys all the elaborate procedures because a very imprecise measure is being used at the end. Unless a measurable outcome criteria can be employed, the trial should not be undertaken.

Tygstrup
I think the question is one of reproducibility, which may be the case with scores but not with clinical impressions.

Blum
By speaking against clinical scores, for clinical judgment, I did not say that we should be satisfied with a hazy clinical judgment. I feel that investigators should clearly try to define what is meant by treatment success or treatment failure, not by making a score, but by defining what they think is better. For example, I can define that an endoscopy is successful when it can be performed within 15 min without the patient gagging, retching, or aspirating. What I object to is giving numbers to these things.

Chalmers
But from this definition a clinical score could now be constructed to evaluate endoscopy.

Lachin
What is important is that a good definition of what constitutes success will lead to consistent scores, and the process of constructing a score often leads to a clarification of the clinical elements which constitute success.

Riis
Our experience is that clinicians are much more aware of the components of so-called clinical judgment when they try to think along these lines. To pinpoint the components of clinical judgments is a positive thing, but we should try to keep the very elaborate statistical methods out of it.

I think these are important considerations because often measurable criteria just are not possible. Consider the evaluation of the quality of life of the patients. Even if there is an exact measure of the effect of treatment, it is equally important to know whether the patient thinks the treatment is worthwhile. Often there will be good agreement between the objective measurements and the patient's feelings, but not always. Nevertheless, I believe that the patient's judgment should be included in the final evaluation.

Tygstrup
I am in favor of quantification, but we should not lose sight of relevance. The aim is to improve the well-being of the patient. If this can be quantified, then fine. Couldn't we agree that relevance comes first and quantification comes soon afterward?

Dropouts and Withdrawals

Lachin
I would like to elaborate on the issue of dropouts and noncompliers. It is a general rule that once a patient is randomized into a treatment

group, he is considered a member of that treatment group in all analyses. In Figure 6.4 there is a normal patient and an alcoholic in each of the two treatment groups. The alcoholic in the placebo group is a noncomplier, a dropout. If he is excluded from the analysis, one group with an alcoholic is being compared to another group where there is no alcoholic. In effect the randomization is destroyed, the groups are no longer comparable, and the comparison is invalid. Patients, therefore, should be included in the group to which they are randomized.

Another point is that in these illustrations it is assumed that an evaluation of outcome was still obtained for the dropouts. In many cases this is not so. Dropouts, however, should still be included in the analyses and an attempt made statistically to evaluate the possible effects of dropouts. One approach is to use a life table analysis in which each patient is included in the analysis over the period of time he or she participated in the trial. But this does not completely eliminate the possibility of bias. The most conservative approach is to simply include all randomized patients in the analysis.

Not all premature exits, however, are dropouts. Figure 6.2 describes the case in which a patient is terminated from therapy due to side effects. Such patients are classified as withdrawals, as described in Chapter 4. Technically this patient is not a dropout; he has reached his outcome. Such events would then be described in separate analyses of side effects.

Finally, the issue of keeping dropouts in the analysis can also be viewed as a clinical issue rather than just statistical. When a physician prescribes a therapy, what is needed is knowledge of the success rate in all those patients for whom the therapy is prescribed--not just for those who take their pills for the full treatment duration. This is the question answered when dropouts are retained.

REFERENCES

1. Peter, P., Bron, B., Kregs, G. J., Pelloni, S., Brandli, H. H., and Blum, A., Kontrollierte studien zur pramedikation von oberen Fiberendoskopien. Zietsch. Gastroenterologien, 1978, 16, 66-72.

2. The Veterans Administration Cooperative Urological Research Group, Treatment and survival of patients with cancer of the prostate. Surg. Gyn. Obstet., 1972, 124, 1011-1017.

3. Best, R. B., Bectel, J. M., and Singleton, J. W., Rederived values of the eight coefficients of the Crohn's disease activity index (CDA). Gastroenterology, 1979, 77, 843-846.

4. Summers, R. W., Switz, D. M., Sessions, J. T., Bectel, J. M., Best, W. R., Kern, F., and Singleton, J. W., National Cooperative Crohn's Disease Study: Results of drug treatment. Gastroenterology, 1979, 77, 847-869.

Part III
Statistical Fundamentals of the Randomized Clinical Trial

7
Statistical Elements of the Randomized Clinical Trial

JOHN M. LACHIN
The George Washington University
Washington, D.C.

7.1 THE CLINICAL TRIAL

A clinical trial can be defined as any prospective controlled assessment of a treatment method, diagnostic technique, or preventive measure. This definition has two key phrases. First is that the trial be prospective, meaning that a cohort, or group of patients, be established who are followed over a period of time and then evaluated with respect to some outcome. Second, the trial should be controlled: it should consist of two or more groups of patients established such that they are comparable with respect to all factors of relevance to the outcomes being assessed.

Sir Bradford Hill, considered by many to be the father of the randomized clinical trial, has said that the essence of the controlled trial is comparison (1). Comparison of the effects of one treatment with another, under conditions in which all other possible intervening factors are accounted for. Thus, at minimum, there should be two groups of patients selected, observed, treated, and evaluated in the same way except for the differences in therapy, not only using the same procedures, but also simultaneously.

This chapter provides an overview of the statistical elements of a clinical trial as they relate to the overall objective, comparison. This is followed by additional chapters which review some of these topics in greater detail.

Clinical trials have essentially three stages: design, execution, and analysis. It is often noted, however, that in many projects the statistician is not consulted until the very end of the study, at the analysis stage. Sometimes it is felt that the statistician causes too much trouble if consulted in the early stages of the study.

The reason for the involvement of the statistician at the earliest stage is that the slightest error in design logic or execution, or failure to adhere to the general overall plan, can have drastic consequences on the methods of analysis employed or the validity of the conclusions drawn, or both. Thus the statistician has largely assumed responsibility for overseeing all the elements of the trial and has considerable contributions to make at each stage. Statisticians have contributed to the development of a number of principles, largely based on scientific logic, which are brought to bear at each stage to ensure the overall scientific integrity of the trial. These principles will be discussed as they relate to each stage of the clinical trial.

7.2 DESIGN
Objectives

The first step in any study is to specify the study design or the overall plan for the study. The development of the design should always start with the goals of the trial, usually presented in terms of conclusions to be reached or hypotheses to be tested. Some considerations in defining these objectives are that

1. The objectives should be <u>realistic</u>. No single clinical trial should be expected to answer all questions of relevance to a given therapy; it is simply impossible. Only those objectives most

relevant to the therapy at the current stage of its testing and development should be considered.
2. The objectives should be <u>in harmony</u> with each other so that all could reasonably be answered with a single overall plan.
3. The objectives should be stated specifically such that they automatically <u>define the outcome events and measures</u> to be employed in the evaluation of the overall success of the study, that is, the dependent variables to be used in the final analyses.

All other design elements are then based on the statement of objectives.

Exclusion Criteria

The study population should then be defined in terms of criteria for patient selection and exclusion, or simply, the exclusion criteria. This should be done with the following in mind.

1. In any clinical trial the welfare of the individual patient should be the foremost consideration. Any patient for whom the therapy might be suspected of posing an additional clinically meaningful risk should be excluded. For this reason most females of childbearing age are usually excluded in a preliminary study of a new drug. This implies in the broader sense that "patients should not be admitted who cannot without hesitation be assigned to any of the study therapies by all of the participating physicians. To do otherwise is ethically inappropriate and scientifically undesirable" (2).
2. Any patient who already manifests an outcome event for the trial should be excluded. For example, in a study of a potentially hepatotoxic agent, toxicity might be evaluated primarily through liver function tests. Thus, patients with known liver disease or pretreatment elevated tests should be excluded because their condition would either mask a mild treatment effect or if their

condition worsened, would defy judgment as to whether the outcome was treatment related.

3. The selection criteria should allow for the evaluation of the objectives with respect to the population at large for whom the treatment is indicated or relevant. That is, these criteria should allow the conclusions reached to be generalized to the general population of interest.

4. To the extent that this does not conflict with the generalization of the results, patients should be excluded who are considered unlikely to complete the period of follow-up for reasons other than potential complications of treatment or the target disease.

Exclusion criteria also have effects on the study in other ways, most notably through Lasagna's law (3) which states that the quickest way to reduce the prevalence of a disease is to study it; as soon as the trial starts, the potential pool of patients available for the study drops significantly. The obvious reason for this in most cases is the exclusion criteria. The exclusion criteria were either too strict or too unrealistic, and the trial was doomed to failure before it even started.

Control Group

It should by now be clear that the description of the effects of treatment is only complete if they are compared to the effects of a control treatment. The purpose of controls, therefore, is to allow the evaluation of the outcomes of interest in a comparable group of patients who receive a standard or best available relevant alternative treatment. There are two key words here, one is relevant and the other is comparable.

1. Relevant means that the same outcome measures used to evaluate the treated group are relevant to the evaluation of the control group. For example, a study of the dissolution of gallstones by chemical means would not use a control group randomized to

undergo gallbladder surgery. The measures used to evaluate the outcome of surgery are different from those one would use for chemical therapy.

2. <u>Comparable</u> means that the patients should not differ in any characteristics, known or unknown, relevant to the outcomes of interest other than the treatment employed.

Randomization

Of all the methods known to the statistician for inducing comparability between groups, randomization is by far the best. There are many methods for randomization (see Chapter 8), but in essence it entails that the treatment of the next patient to enter the trial is determined purely by chance, and not by any characteristics of the patient. This ensures that characteristics known or unknown did not influence the treatment assigned, thus promoting comparability of the study groups.

Statistically, randomization does two things. First, it eliminates sources of incomparability in that it controls the probability that the groups will differ on any characteristic by more than some specified relative amount. Further, as the sample size to be used in the study is increased, the probability that the groups will differ by this amount approaches zero. This probability can be assessed by the simple equation

$$p = 2[1 - \Phi(y)]$$

where

$$y = \frac{\delta \sqrt{n}}{\sqrt{2\pi(1-\pi)}}$$

δ = degree of imbalance
π = prevalence of the characteristic in the population
n = sample size per group
Φ = normal distribution probability function;
    e.g., $\Phi(1.645) = 0.95$

For example, suppose there is a relevant characteristic observed in 40% of all the patients in the population ($\pi = 0.40$). Two hundred patients are then randomized to each group (n = 200), and it is hoped that 40% of the patients in both groups a and b will have this characteristic, meaning that they will be equally balanced. We will, however, be willing to tolerate some imbalance. From this equation, the probability of having an imbalance of say 20% ($\delta = 0.20$), such as 30% in one group and 50% in the other group, where the two groups each have 200 patients, is less than 1 in 40,000 ($p \leq 0.000024$).

Thus randomization allows the computation of the probability that these groups will differ by a specified amount, not only for the characteristics known but also for the characteristics unknown. Randomization does not explicitly guarantee perfect comparability of the groups with respect to characteristics of interest, it promotes it, and promotes it better than any other known procedure.

Second, randomization allows a standard statistical test of significance to be conducted. I consider this, however, to be a secondary argument for randomization. What is important is that the correct conclusion be reached scientifically, and for this I consider randomization to be essential, not only for the statistical justification of the significance test, but in terms of scientific comparison being the main objective.

Randomization may be <u>restricted or unrestricted</u>, with each procedure for restricted randomization necessitating a different form of analysis. The most common restrictions are stratification and pairing. These restrictions may also be used in conjunction with more sophisticated experimental designs, however, the following considers only the simple group comparison design as explained in Chapter 4.

Stratification

In stratified randomization (prospective stratification), one or more characteristics are defined which are known beforehand to be related to the outcomes of interest, and then a series of strata or groups of patients are defined based on these characteristics. Patients are then randomized within the strata to which they belong. Consider a study in which it is known that the patients of different ages and sex have differing prognosis. It might be decided to stratify on these two variables by defining four separate randomization plans, one each for the young males, the young females, the old males, and the old females. Since each patient is randomized within his or her stratum we are assured a good balance between the treatments within each of these strata, and thus we are assured a good balance between these strata within each treatment.

Further, there are two ways to stratify prospectively. One is to specify beforehand the sample size in each stratum. For example, it might be desired to study 20 patients in each stratum. Patients then would be recruited until each of the four strata of 20 patients had been filled. Another method of stratification would simply be to use open-ended randomization lists whereby each patient would be randomized according to the list for the stratum to which he or she belongs, with no restrictions on the size of the strata. This in turn might entail a different method of analysis, since the strata will likely have different numbers of patients.

I should confess at this point that I consider stratified randomization to be of value only in cases in which there is going to be a small overall sample size. There are two reasons for this. First, as was pointed out earlier, randomization by itself is highly effective, especially when one is dealing with sample sizes of 100 or more patients per group. Second, if any imbalance does occur, there are methods for the analysis of the data based on retrospective postrandomization stratification which would account for any imbalances observed, unlikely as they are.

A related issue, often confused with stratification, is where it is desired to ensure that a specified percentage of the study patients either have or do not have a certain characteristic. In this case it is recommended that a quota system be adopted rather than employ stratified randomization. For example, it might be desired to restrict obese patients to comprise no more than 25% of the study sample. Rather than establish a separate stratum in this case, a quota system would be just as effective as stratification and easier to implement. Under a quota system, obese patients would be eligible for randomization, using a single randomization plan for all subjects, until the quota, 25% of the total projected sample size, was filled. The data could then be analyzed using postrandomization stratification on the quota variables.

Matching or Pairing

The second form of restricted randomization often used is matching or pairing, whereby patients are randomized in matched-pairs, each pair of patients being matched according to one or more specified characteristics. Upon randomization, the members of each pair are randomly assigned one to each treatment group. Patient-matching is most feasible when all patients, or the great majority, are known before the study starts. Otherwise, if patients are recruited slowly, the inability to construct pairs and randomize them rapidly reduces the overall numbers of patients available to the study. Thus, patient-matching is most beneficial when a small total sample is required and the patients are known beforehand.

The pair, however, need not consist of two patients. A natural form of pairing is commonly employed in ophthalmologic studies wherein a pair of diseased eyes is the sampling unit, as with studies of diabetic retinopathy. A patient with disease in both eyes is recruited and each eye randomly assigned to receive either of two therapies.

Another form of pairing is the collection of repeated or serial measurements on each patient. Thus the crossover design (see Chapter 12) is a special case of pairing.

If pairing is employed, the outcome must be carefully defined because all patient pairs may not contribute equally to the analysis. For example, for a discrete, binary (+, -) outcome, most methods of analysis use only the discordant pairs, i.e., the pairs in which one but not both members are a success (i.e., +- or -+). The pairs in which both patients are treatment successes (++) or both patients treatment failures (--) do not enter into the analysis. Thus, it is imperative that most if not all pairs be discordant for both ethical and statistical reasons. This is only achieved with clear objective criteria for declaring treatment a or b better within each pair, such as time to remission.

In summary, the use of a simple randomization plan is recommended, usually without stratification and without patient-matching.

Blinding

A design characteristic frequently mentioned in preceding chapters is blinding or masking. Under a _single blind_, either the patient or the physician knows the treatment which has been assigned, but not both. Under a _double blind_, neither the physician nor the patient are aware of the treatment assigned. The objective of blinding, as with randomization, is to induce comparability in the way that patients are recruited, treated, and observed. Blinding does this in two ways. First, it avoids bias in the evaluation of treatment effects by promoting uniformity in the recruitment, treatment, and observation of all patients. Second, and an important factor often overlooked, blinding preserves the integrity of the randomization. It prevents either the physician (or the patient) from knowingly, actively diverting the patient to a different group from that to which he was (or was to be) randomized. This is an important problem in unblinded or single blind studies.

Trial Period

As was indicated in Chapters 5 and 6, dropouts or noncompliant patients can be a difficult problem in any clinical trial. One way of reducing the extent of this problem is to employ a trial period. In this procedure eligible patients are placed on a short program of therapy using the control (e.g., placebo) medication prior to actual randomization. Noncompliant patients can be detected through pill counts or other means and excluded from the clinical trial prior to randomization. This is important, because once randomized, a patient should be included in all analyses, even if noncompliant. The only possible exceptions are those cases in which a randomized patient is later found not to have met the eligibility criteria due to an error in eligibility screening. This problem can also be minimized, however, by a trial period, because this affords some extra time for a colleague or coordinating center to review the eligibility of all patient candidates while they undergo their trial period.

A related issue is that patients may have their pills analyzed to find out if they are receiving placebo. This often happens in a drug trial and could induce bias since the patients on placebo will likely then drop out while those on active medication will stay in. But if all patients have an initial trial period of placebo therapy (unknown to the patient), then it is likely that the pill analyzers will have their trial period medication analyzed and will complain because it shows they are on placebo. Such patients can be excluded prior to randomization with less chance of bias.

Follow-up Schedule

The next major design feature concerns the schedule of follow-up visits (month 1, 2, and so on), the duration of follow-up, and the exact measurements and procedures to be conducted at each visit or at each point in time. Again, the follow-up schedule should be based on the objectives of the trial, and it should be designed to yield the data required to evaluate the objectives. This is especially important in a multicenter trial in which, in addition, the methodology of all measurements and procedures should be specified thoroughly.

An important statistical feature is that all follow-up visits should be timed in relation to the date of randomization for each patient, and that fairly narrow "windows" be specified for each visit. In the statistical analysis it may be important that the patient experience after, say, 6 months be evaluated, in which case each visit at month 6 should occur within the 30 days defining month 6 for each patient, and not anywhere from months 4 through 8. Thus, the period of follow-up for each patient should be defined in precise time intervals.

Basically, two types of follow-up schedules can be employed. In the first, each patient is treated for a period of <u>fixed maximum length</u>, say, 1 year. Each patient is then treated for only 1 year and then the treatment is terminated. This is the most prevalent type of follow-up schedule and allows the use of relatively straightforward methods of analysis. The trial is concluded when the last randomized patient has reached the end of his or her 1 year of therapy.

In the second type of follow-up schedule, each patient would continue treatment, regardless of how long after randomization, until a specified <u>common end date</u>, such as when the last randomized patient has reached the end of 1 year of therapy. In this case patients will have been treated for various lengths of time, thus requiring that more sophisticated methods of analysis be employed.

Each of these follow-up plans has its own advantages and disadvantages, both operationally and statistically. Consider a study with a 2-year recruitment period and a minimum follow-up of 1 year, a total of 3 years duration. If all patients are treated for only 1 year (fixed length), the patient load in each clinic declines during the last year as only the last patients entered are followed. On the other hand, however, this allows more careful review of data on those patients already treated, so that final analyses can be rapidly initiated at the end of 3 years.

On the other hand, following all patients up to the end of the third year (common end date) maintains a high patient load in each clinic until the end, but leaves little time for careful review of patient data before beginning final analyses, and often analyses are delayed.

Statistically, both plans equally allow evaluation of the effects of therapy after 1 year. The second plan, however, allows evaluation up to 2 years for some of the patients, and 3 years for a few. If the therapy has a long-term therapeutic effect, the statistical difference between treatment versus control might thereby be greater after 3 years of follow-up, increasing the statistical power of the study.

In addition, statistical methods are available to help estimate the optimal length of followup and optimal frequency with which a test or procedure should be repeated during the follow-up period (4).

Clinical Management Procedures

Finally, procedures for the clinical management of suspected disease- or treatment-related complications should be clearly specified, especially in the multicenter trial. Although this is largely a clinical concern, such procedures have important statistical consequences, especially where such complications are to be tabulated as outcome events, as in the evaluation of the toxicity of a new therapy. In such cases the procedures for clinical management should be standardized as much as possible while still being consistent with generally accepted proper clinical practice.

7.3 SAMPLE SIZE

The next statistical issue is the determination of the sample size. Although this is reviewed in greater detail in Chapter 9, I would here like to give an overview of the problem.

Sample Size Determination

In a clinical trial, as in any experiment, one starts out to reach a decision, or in statistical terms an inference, about the true state of nature. But such decisions must be made in the face of variation or uncertainty. Thus, when the trial is designed, there should be a high probability of detecting a minimal, clinically relevant difference, i.e., a difference which would lead to a preference for one therapy over the other in clinical practice (see Chapter 4). The probability of detecting this difference, however, will depend largely on the sample size. If the probability of detecting a relevant difference is small, the trial might as well not be started because the odds are that the results will be negative more often than not.

For example, suppose the efficacy of a new drug is to be tested and it is felt that the treatment should show an increase of at least 10% in the cure rate above that shown by controls, where the control rate is expected to be 20% or less. Thus, 10% is the minimal, clinically relevant difference. Statistically it can be determined that about 320 patients per group are required to yield a 90% chance of detecting a difference of 10% when a statistical test is conducted at the 0.05 significance level (5, 6), (see Chapter 9).

There is often confusion on this point, so let me clarify by explaining what is not being done. This does not mean that if a difference of 10% is obtained in a sample, the study will achieve significance at the 0.05 level with 320 patients per group. What is meant is that if the underlying real difference in the population is 10%, if this is the real description of the treated difference in the population, then with 320 patients in each group the study will have a 90% chance of finding a statistically significant difference. Had the study used only 100 patients per group, it would only have a 50% chance of reaching significance, and so on. Thus, the probability of detecting a relevant difference depends largely on the sample size.

Secondary Objectives--Subgroups

In addition to the clinically relevant difference it is hoped to detect, a number of other factors could affect the sample size requirements. Among the secondary objectives of many clinical trials are subgroup analyses, such as evaluating whether the effect of treatment among males differs from that among females. As a general rule it can be shown that an analysis across subgroups will sometimes require as many as four times the patients required for a simple two-group analysis. Thus, in the above example, if the problem of subgroups were of interest, a sample size as large as 1280 per group might be required, rather than just 320 (5,7).

Multiple Objectives

A related factor is that many clinical trials have multiple objectives, such as safety and efficacy, each of which will require a different sample size. In general, safety (or toxicity) is the most difficult objective to evaluate because it is desired that small differences be detected. Safety can never be "proven," because there is always the possibility of the rare toxic event. In such cases the sample size required should be computed for each objective and that one selected which is most appropriate--cost, resources, and other factors considered.

Now suppose a realistic sample size is chosen which is adequate for some objectives but not all. An alternative approach might be to determine that difference which the study would have a high probability of detecting given the sample size to be used. In a trial in which one of the objectives is the evaluation of toxicity, an objective which will require a vast number of patients, a sample size determination might be developed based on efficacy, and then the toxicity rate determined which the study would have a good chance of detecting with that sample size.

For example, suppose that a statistical test is to be conducted at the 0.05 significance level and the sample size is fixed at 300 patients per group from previous considerations. But it is also desired to have an 80% chance of detecting some toxicity. It can be determined that with this sample size, there will be an 80% chance of detecting a 5% difference when the control side-effect rate does not exceed 1%. This is another way of evaluating the effects of the sample size on the overall outcome of the study.

Dropouts

Another factor with great implications for the adequacy of a sample size and the methods of analysis is the dropout rate. In any trial patients will become dissillusioned or lose interest and simply drop out of the trial. Since it is never certain that such dropping out is <u>not</u> related to the treatment in perhaps subtle ways, all dropouts must be included in the analysis, i.e., in the denominator when computing the proportions of successes or failures. Thus, in the analysis of the data there is a general rule that once a patient has been randomized to a treatment group, the patient is considered a member of that group regardless of any other outcome. This includes patients who do not adhere to the therapy, patients who fail to complete the period of follow-up for any reason, patients who do not achieve full dosage in a variable dosage plan, and so on. If the dropouts are eliminated from the sample, one may very well be left with two incompletely randomized groups, which may be incomparable with respect to one or more factors of interest, especially if dropping out is related to the treatment. For this reason dropouts should be included in all subsequent analyses. But when doing so, any treatment effects which might exist are diluted, and as a result, a larger sample size will be needed to detect a difference of a given magnitude.

A general rule is expressed in the simple equation $N_d = N/(1 - R)^2$, where N_d is the sample size with an R% dropout rate, and N is the sample size without dropouts (5). For example, for a 30% dropout rate (R = 0.30), the sample size must be doubled in order to have the same probability of detecting a difference as one would have without dropouts. For this reason, care must be taken when conducting or analyzing a trial with a dropout rate exceeding 15%.

Unbalanced Designs

Any trial with unequal sample sizes in the treatment groups is called an unbalanced design. While some slight imbalance may result from the randomization process itself, it is the planned imbalance which is referred to, such as when there are twice as many patients in the treated group as placebo. While such designs may have an advantage in some situations, I have generally not found them to be advantageous in clinical trials, mainly due to the multiplicity of objectives. Overall it has been suggested that the most efficient design, statistically, is to use equal-sized treatment groups, even when using more than two groups (8).

7.4 EXECUTION

The quality of any clinical trial lies in many considerations other than its basic design. The most well designed clinical trial is worthless unless it is properly executed. Although many of the following points will be elaborated in later chapters, I would like to here review those aspects of execution which have traditionally become the statistican's responsibility.

Forms Design

In the final evaluation of any trial, the results of the trial and the statistical analyses will only be as good, as sound, and as precise as the data obtained on the study forms. In a small trial the study forms may be as simple as a single standardized data sheet; or in a large-scale multicenter trial, there may be numerous study forms, each to be completed in a given situation. In either case it must be remembered that if the data were not properly collected on the study forms they will not be available for anlaysis. Thus, the development of the study forms requires careful consideration and collaboration among the statisticians and clinicians involved.

Computerization

The next step is to computerize these study forms. By this I mean to organize the study forms into a data base which can be augmented as additional information on each patient becomes available, and which can be used as a basis for the statistical analyses. For a large-scale trial, sophisticated data base management techniques will be required, and in my view, the adequacy of these data management systems is perhaps one of the most critical aspects in trial execution. There are two crucial considerations here:

1. It should be understood, especially in the large multicenter trial, that highly capable technical support by systems analysts and programmers will be required to make the whole system work. The statistician should not be expected to provide this level of technical support since it is very rare that a statistician is able to acquire a high degree of competence in both statistics and computer science.

2. It should also be understood that despite its image, the computer is not capable of all wonders. It is a common misconception that once the data has been "computerized," the computer can spit it back upon demand. In many large-scale trials, the data base management procedures are so sophisticated that such an instantaneous response is simply not feasible. Of course, if desired, it would be possible to develop such a system, but at great cost.

All participants, therefore, should approach the computerized data systems with professional respect and a realistic expectation of what will be its capabilities and limitations.

Editing

Among the important aspects of a computerized data management system is the facility for data-editing. By this is meant checking to see if a given data item is within an acceptable range, or is missing, or whether it is consistent with other items on the data form or other data forms received previously. The objective is to detect errors so that they can be corrected quickly rather than at the end of the trial when the data analysis is conducted. Again, the needs for such editing vary depending on the scope of the trial, but for a large multicenter trial, extensive data-editing procedures will be required. In conjunction with these procedures, a system to distribute error notices to the participating clinics and to post corrections against the computerized files will be necessary.

Quality Control

This leads to the general issue of quality control in clinical trials. In a multicenter trial it is important that every unit of the organization, the treatment centers, central laboratories if any, central reading units, and the actual statistical support center be quality controlled. Although data-editing is an important aspect of this process, it should not stop here. Some clinical trials have found site visits to be a very helpful mechanism. For example, in a large-scale trial, a standing monitoring team might be established for each of the central units, including the statistical support center. The site visit team would consist of people with appropriate expertise who would visit the respective unit on a periodic basis to review procedures and to make recommendations for improvements in these procedures. Again, the overall objective is to ensure the integrity of the trial by maximizing the accuracy with which the protocol is executed.

7.5 ETHICS

Much has been written about the ethics of the randomized clinical trial, and I will not attempt in any way to cover all the issues. Some of these issues, however, relate directly to the needs for data analysis, and it is within this context that I think it appropriate to discuss ethics.

Much of my views on these matters have been based on the writings of Larry Shaw and Tom Chalmers (2) (see also Ref. 9), and I strongly encourage all clinical trials participants to review these important papers. Briefly, they consider randomization to be the appropriate course whenever doubt exists as to the superiority of one therapy over another. By randomizing, each patient entering the trial then has an equal chance of receiving whichever therapy eventually may be proven to be the therapy of choice. Of course, whenever it is known that one of the two therapies under consideration is superior, it is ethically required that the trial be stopped and the superior therapy be made available to all study participants. Thus, it is ethically required that the accumulating results be reviewed as the trial progresses.

Shaw and Chalmers also point out that the individual study physicians should be blinded to the accumulating data because the ethics of their participation in the trial might be influenced by a "trend" which suggests, but does not prove, the superiority of one therapy over another. Thus, they recommend that interim data analyses be conducted on a periodic basis which are reviewed by a data-monitoring committee. Only when this committee observes that the superiority for one therapy is statistically proven should the trial be stopped and the results disclosed to the general scientific community.

7.6 ANALYSIS

Interim Analyses

Interim analyses of accumulating data, however, pose many methodological problems, the most important being termed sampling to

<u>a foregone conclusion</u>. Most standard methods of statistical analysis (e.g., chi-square tests, t-tests) are based on the assumption that the sample size to be used is fixed and that the data will be analyzed only once, at the end of the study. Thus, the repeated analysis of accumulating data, as in the interim analyses for a clinical trial, violates this critical assumption. As a result, each time these standard statistical methods might be naively applied, there would be an increasing chance that the data would show "significance" even though there might be no real difference between the two therapies. It can be shown mathematically that sooner or later with certainty such a significant result would be reached if the trial were to continue indefinitely. Thus the phrase sampling to a foregone conclusion, (see Ref. 10.).

Interim analyses, therefore, require a different approach from those standard methods which might be employed in the final analyses. This problem has received much attention and adequate statistical methods for such interim analyses are available (see Ref. 11). Reveiw of these methods is given in Chapter 11.

Multiple Variables

A related problem concerns the multiplicity of dependent variables. The same type of problem which occurs with repeated sequential looks also occurs when there are many dependent variables. Sooner or later some of these will show significance by chance alone. For this reason the outcomes to be used in both the interim and final analyses should be clearly defined beforehand, and where possible appropriate statistical techniques employed to minimize the problems involved with multiple dependent variables.

Dropouts

Another common methodological problem is the presence of dropouts. For reasons explained above, dropouts should be included in the analysis.

Statistical Elements   97

There are many ways to do this. One would be to simply include the dropouts in all denominators, and in the numerators if they had incurred an event, when computing simple proportions. This, however, ignores the differential period of follow-up for dropouts and nondropouts. Another method of analysis is to use the life table method, which is adequate primarily when the dropouts probably are not related to the treatment, but this is very difficult to prove.

The Life Table Method

One of the most important methods of analysis developed for clinical trials is the life table method, so called because the analysis examines the experience (life) of the cohort over the various periods of followup in the same way mortality experience is analyzed in a life table, (see Refs. 12 and 13). This method is especially useful in trials in which patients are followed for differing lengths of time, e.g., some patients drop out or terminate therapy prematurely for disease-or treatment-related complications, or all patients are followed to a common end date. In a life table analysis each patient is counted in the analysis for the period over which he or she was followed and observed, i.e., was at risk for an event. Such an analysis, therefore, requires that the period of follow-up for each patient be defined in precise time intervals.

Subgroup Analyses

Another analytic issue is the use of subgroup analyses to attempt to identify intervening factors which might be of relevance to the outcome, either treatment success or the development of side effects. In addition to the problem of multiplicity of analyses, this often raises the problem of post hoc analyses, i.e., an analysis conducted after observing the data, an analysis that had not been planned originally but is suggested by the data itself. Such analyses are often called "fishing expeditions" and are made possible because the data often include information about a multitude of possibly prognostic factors, not just those suspected on the basis of previous studies. Such analyses are often very useful, but should be approached with caution.

The life table method and subgroup comparisons are described in greater detail in Chapter II.

Prediction

One reasonable method of analysis which has often been neglected in clinical trials is the use of ancillary data in an attempt at prediction, predicting the risk factors for treatment failure or predicting the prognostic factors for treatment success. Methods exist for employing such data in mathematical models which can be applied to future patients. If properly developed and validated, such predictive models would allow the evaluation of the prognosis for a future patient based on that patient's characteristics. An outstanding example of this approach was the identification of cholesterol level and smoking history, among other characteristics, as predictors of cardiovascular events (14).

In conclusion, the statistical elements of the clinical trial are all summarized in the statement that <u>every activity</u> undertaken during a trial has real or potential implications for either the methods of analysis, or the validity of the conclusions drawn, or both.

7.7 DISCUSSION
Stratification

<u>Schoenfield</u>
A plea was made for randomization with as little stratification as possible. Suppose that it is known from a previous study that a particular variable will indeed influence the results. In that instance would stratification be recommended?

<u>Lachin</u>
Only if the sample size is small enough that it could readily lead to an imbalance which, though small in absolute numbers, might nevertheless affect the outcome of the study. There has been much controversy about the value of stratification and the concensus is that stratification is helpful with small sample sizes. For larger sample sizes it doesn't

hurt, but it has not been shown to definitely help either. The reason I do not advocate stratification for larger sample sizes is because it causes many additional administrative problems. In many of the studies in which the randomization has gone bad, it was due to errors related to stratification; i.e., patients were randomized using the randomization schedule for the wrong strata. In other words, a young male might have been randomized according to the old male randomization plan.

Tygstrup
You say that stratification will not hurt, but I think it may because the trial is broken down into a number of smaller trials, each of which has its own requirements for sample size, and so it may increase the probability of a type II error.

Lachin
That is true if the analyses within every one of the stratum are a primary aim of the study, but not if the objective is simply to facilitate the comparability of the two groups.

In my opinion the design of any study should be as simple as possible. Stratification should be avoided unless it is absolutely necessary. There are many reasons for this; one is the ability to adjust for other factors in the analysis, but more important is the execution of the study. The simpler the design the easier it will be to execute the study and the less the possibility for error.

Chalmers
This points out that we are talking about an extremely complex phenomenon in which the physician must spend a lot of time with the biostatistician, discussing the pros and cons of one maneuver or another to finally end up with the best compromise possible. Every clinical trial is a compromise with the available techniques.

Dropouts versus Withdrawals

Student
Is a dropout the same as a patient who is withdrawn from therapy due to complications?

Lachin
In general, statisticians refer not just to dropouts but to censored observations, dropping out being one major reason for censoring. A censored observation is any patient who does not complete the prescribed period of therapy and is not evaluated with respect to the outcome of interest to be evaluated. The important key phrase here is that the patient is not evaluated with respect to the outcome of interest.

There are many different outcomes in a clinical trial. For example, consider a study of the efficacy and safety of a drug treatment with potential side effects. Each patient is to be treated for

2 years. Now suppose a patient is terminated from therapy due to a drug-related reaction after 9 months. The patient, therefore, is a treatment failure, or what we have called a withdrawal, and would contribute fully to the analyses of side-effect rates. The patient, however, was only exposed to therapy for 9 months and would be handled as a censored observation in the analyses of the 2-year efficacy rate. In this latter respect, this patient is equivalent to a patient who just dropped out at 9 months. The strict dropout, the patient who refuses to continue, however, is different, since that patient would not contribute outcome data to any analysis, neither that of efficacy nor that of safety.

In general, therefore, we should speak of the broad class of censored observations, what have been called exits from study, rather than just dropouts who strictly speaking are the patients who cease participation for reasons other than effects of the target disease or therapy. The important point, however, is that a given patient may be considered a censored observation in one analysis but not another, it depends on the outcome being evaluated.

Riis
But not all patients who do not complete the period of therapy are censored because of dropping out or side effects. In some studies a patient's therapy is stopped early if he or she reaches success with therapy. You know the complete answer for this patient and he should not be confused with dropouts.

Lachin
That is true, but a premature treatment success is also an exit from study and would be treated as a censored observation in analyses of short-term toxicity since that patient would no longer be at risk of a drug-related side effect. For long-term toxicity, e.g., a delayed toxic reaction, however, that patient would be censored when last observed, which might be long after having been healed.

Unbalanced Designs

Schoenfield
In the discussion of unbalanced designs, what would be recommended when there are three groups, one a placebo group, and two treatments which are in fact a high dose and a low dose of the same drug? What should be the distribution of patients in these three groups? Should it be 1:1:1 or perhaps 1 in the placebo group to each 1 in the other groups, i.e., 2:1:1.

Juhl
On the basis of ethical considerations each patient should have equal chance of getting the active therapy, i.e., 2:1:1.

Schoenfield
This is an interesting point: there are two reasons often considered for having a larger number of patients in the placebo group than in the treatment groups. One reason is that we may not want a patient to feel he has a 2:1 chance of receiving therapy. One argument against that, however, might be that the low-dose therapy is suboptimal for which there is not yet evidence for efficacy. Often such a low dose is employed to help evaluate a dose relationship to toxicity.

The other reason is the widely employed statistical rule that if a placebo group is compared against K treatment groups, the allocation to placebo should be proportional to the square root of K for each patient assigned to active treatment, i.e., 1.4 to placebo for each 1 in the treated groups in a three-group trial. I know this is applied when comparing one placebo with two different treatments, but does the same figure apply when comparing placebo to two doses of the same agent?

Lachin
The square root rule is based on the Dunnett (15) procedure for conducting a separate t-test comparing each treatment group against the control group such that the overall type I error does not exceed the desired α level. Dunnett showed that the power of the paired comparisons are maximized when the ratio of the sample size for placebo to that of each of the other groups satisfies the square root rule. Thus, the rule applies for multiple drugs versus placebo or multiple doses versus placebo.

This procedure, however, is based upon the concept of paired comparisons using a quantitative measure, and not upon the overall comparison of the treatments. Usually in a clinical trial the outcome is qualitative, e.g., the percentage of success, and in this example, a 2 x 3 chi-square test would be used for the overall comparison of the three groups. Now in this case the question is whether an imbalance in the sample allocations affects the overall chi-square test. Here the square root rule does not apply. Sometimes the optimal sample allocation to placebo which will maximize the power of the chi-square test is greater than 1 in 3 and sometimes it is less than 1 in 3; it depends upon the simultaneous differences among the three groups which it is desired to detect. Thus, when an overall comparison of all groups is to be conducted, I feel that the best procedure is to use equal sample allocations because this tends to maximize the average power over the tests to be conducted for the various outcomes (7).

This, however, is a statistical argument, not an ethical one. If the clinicians then decide that the ethical argument outweighs the statistical, the sample size should be calculated with that in mind.

REFERENCES

1. Hill, A. B., Controlled Clinical Trials, Balckwell, Oxford, 1960.
2. Shaw, L. W., and Chalmers, T. C., Ethics in cooperative clinical trials. Ann. N.Y. Acad. Sci., 1970, 169, 487-489.
3. Gorringe, J. A. L., Initial preparation for clinical trials, in The Principles and Practice of Clinical Trials (E. L. Harris and J. D. Fitzgerald, eds.), E & S Livingstone, Edinburg and London, 1970, pp. 41-46.
4. Schlesselman , J., Planning a longitudinal study: II. Frequency of measurement and study duration. J. Chron. Dis., 1973, 26, 561-570.
5. Lachin, J. M., An introduction to sample size determination and power analysis for clinical trials. Controlled Clinical Trials, 1981, 2, 93-113.
6. Lachin, J.M., M., Sample size considerations for clinical trials of potentially hepatotoxic drugs, in Guidelines for Detection of Heaptotoxicity Due to Drugs and Chemicals, C. S. Davidson, C. M. Leevy, and E. C. Chamberlayne, eds.), U.S. Department of H.E.W., National Institutes of Health, NIH Publication No. 79-313, 1979, pp. 119-130.
7. Lachin, J. M., Marks, J. W., Schoenfield, L.J., and the NCGS Protocol Committee and the National Cooperative Gallstone Study Group, Design and methodological considerations in the National Cooperative Gallstone Study: A multicenter clinical trial. Controlled Clinical Trials, 1981, 2, 177-230.
8. Lachin, J. M., Sample size determination for r x c comparative trials. Biometrics, 1977, 33, 315-324.
9. Chalmers, T., Ethical aspects of clinical trials. Amer. J. Opthalmology, 1975, 79, 753-758.
10. McPherson, K., Statistics: The problem of examining accumulating data more than once. N. Engl. J. Med. 1974, 290, 501-502.
11. Armitage, P., Sequential Medical Trials, Wiley, New York, 1975.
12. Cutler, S. J., and Ederer, F., Maximum utilization of the life table method in analyzing survival. J. Chron. Dis., 1958, 8, 699-712.
13. Peto, R., Pike, M. C., Armitage, P., Breslow, N. E., Cox, D. R., Howard, S. V., Mantel, N., McPherson, K., Peto, J., and Smith, P. G., Design and analysis of randomized clinical trials requiring prolonged observation of each patient: II. Analysis and examples. Brit. J. Cancer, 1977, 35, 1-39.

14. Truett, J., Cornfield, J., and Kannel, W., A multivariate analysis of the risk of coronary heart disease in Framingham. J. Chron. Dis., 1967, 20, 511-524.

15. Dunnett, C. W., A multiple comparison procedure for comparing several treatments with a control. J. Amer. Stat. Ass., 1955, 50, 1096-1121.

ADDITIONAL READINGS

Brown, B. W., Statistical controversies in the design of clinical trials--some personal views. Controlled Clinical Trials, 1980, 1, 13-28.

Cornfield, J., Recent methodological contributions to clinical trials. Amer. J. Epidemiol., 1976, 104, 408-421.

Cox, D. R., Planning of Experiments, Wiley, New York, 1958.

Ederer, F., Patient bias, investigator bias and the double masked procedure in clinical trials. Amer. J. Med., 1975, 58, 295-299.

Ederer, F., The statistician's role in developing a protocol for a clinical trial. American Statistician, 1979, 33, 116-119.

Feinstein, A. R., Clinical Biostatistics, C. V. Mosby, St. Louis, Mo., 1977.

Forster, F. M. (ed.) Evaluation of Drug Therapy, the University of Wisconsin Press, Madison, Wis., 1961.

Harris, E. L. and Fitzgerald, S. D. (eds.), The Principles and Practice of Clinical Trials, Livingstone, Edinburg and London, 1970.

Mantel, N., A miscellany of statistical and other considerations for clinical trials, Controlled Clinical Trials, 1980, 1, 3-12.

Meier, P., Statistics and medical experimentation. Biometrics, 1975, 31, 511-529.

Mosteller, F., Gilbert, J. P. and McPeek, B. Reporting standards and research strategies for controlled trials: Agenda for the editor. Controlled Clinical Trials, 1980, 1, 37-58.

Peto, R., Pike, M. C., Armitage, P., Breslow, N. E., Cox, D. R., Howard, S. V., Mantel, N., McPherson, K., Peto, J. and Smith, P. G. Design and analysis of randomized clinical trials requiring prolonged observation of each patient: I. Introduction and design. Brit. J. Cancer, 1976, 34, 585-612.

Shaw, L. W., Cornfield, J. and Cole, C. M., Statistical problems in the design of clinical trials and interpretation of results, in Thrombosis: Pathogenesis and Clinical Trials (E. Deutsch, K. M. Brinkhous, K. Lechner, and S. Hinnom, eds.), F. K. Schattauer Verlay, Stuttgart and New York, 1973, pp. 191-202.

Schwartz, D., and Lellouch, J., Explanatory and pragmatic attitudes in therapeutic trials. J. Chron. Dis., 1967, 20, 637-648.

8
Why Randomization Is Essential and How to Do It

AVIVA PETRIE*
London School of Hygiene and Tropical Medicine
and Royal Postgraduate Medical School
London, England

8.1 WHY WE RANDOMIZE

"Somewhere between 1910 and 1912 in this country, a random patient, with a random disease, consulting a doctor chosen at random, had, for the first time in the history of mankind, a better than fifty-fifty chance of profitering from the encounter!" This quotation of Lawrence J. Henderson (1878-1932) in the New England Journal of Medicine (1) perhaps mocks the process in which statisticians place so much faith, the process of randomization. However, all things in moderation!

    Randomization fulfills a useful, and to the majority, essential role in the design and resulting validity of a clinical trial. It would seem, though, that we have to clarify the meaning of the term randomization. A set of treatments applied to a set of individuals is said to be randomized when the treatment applied to any given individual is chosen at random (by chance methods) from those available. Our concern is with randomizing the treatments.

---

*Ms. Petrie is currently with the London School of Hygiene and Tropical Medicine, London, England.

Why is this randomization process essential? To what end is it performed? Basically, there are three main reasons for randomization. First, and this perhaps is the most obvious reason, randomization enables the removal of differences in the characteristics exhibited by the groups receiving the various treatments. These characteristics may influence response to treatment. Thus, this attempt to achieve homogeneity of these characteristics among the groups goes far to alleviate bias in the results. Two examples of characteristics which typically influence response to treatment are sex and age. By randomizing the treatments to the patients, it is probable that the treatment groups will be alike in all respects other than the treatments the individuals in these groups receive, whether or not the characteristics influencing response are known in advance. Chapter 7 has already described how to actually calculate the probability that two randomized groups will differ by a stated amount on any characteristic.

A second reason for randomization is to enable statistical sampling theory to apply. It should be remembered that when a clinical trial is performed on a set of individuals, these individuals are, in reality, a sample of individuals selected from a population of individuals. Sampling theory forms the basis for statistical tests and estimation procedures.

Finally, randomization permits concealment (i.e., blinding) of the identity of the treatment either from the physician or from the patient or from them both. Blinding may be important in removing bias when the assessment of response is subjective. Randomization does not ensure blinding, but it is difficult to arrange any form of blinding without randomization. Thus, randomization is a necessary although not sufficient condition for blinding.

An added advantage of randomization which is seldom voiced might be termed political. When a conclusion is reached as to the efficacy or toxicity of a new treatment, those conducting the trial must present their results in a credible fashion to the rest of the community.

The absence of randomization detracts from this credibility, particularly when the conclusions are unexpected or unwarranted, and the value of the trial can be substantially undermined.

It would seem, thus far, that randomization presents no problem and must surely be employed in all clinical trials. Why, then, the controversy, which most certainly exists? The fundamental dilemma of randomization arises from the conflict between the individual patient and the scientific concept of medicine. Is priority to be given to administering the best treatment to the patient at hand or to the acquisition of knowledge for use in the future treatment of a hypothetical patient population? The debate will continue and will probably remain a topic of controversy for many years to come. Certainly there are situations in which we may question the advisability of randomization, but in general, I find it hard to doubt its efficacy and ethical feasibility.

As a potential patient, I remain impervious to the uncertainties suggested by the dilemma. It is a generally accepted condition that a clinical trial should not be conducted unless the trial is ethically justified. This being so, the physician involved must initially have an "agnostic" attitude as to the relative merits of the alternative treatments. In these circumstances, the conflict of the dilemma is not of issue.

Before rushing headlong into the practicalities of randomization, some mention should be made of the disadvantages inherent in the technique. Foremost, perhaps, is its effect of undermining the doctor-patient relationship. It is difficult for the patient to place implicit trust in the doctor when the doctor, in order to satisfy ethical considerations, admits to an agnostic attitude as to the relative merits of the treatments. Surely some faith in the healer must be destroyed if the healer is not sure of how best to heal?

A second problem with randomization is that it can go bad; in particular, it may not fully remove differences in the characteristics exhibited by the groups receiving the different treatments. This is a chance phenomenon unlikely to occur if the sample size is sufficiently large. It is a hazard we are generally prepared to accept. Finally, the randomization procedure itself may be rather cumbersome, but this is a small price to pay for the advantages proffered.

8.2 HOW TO RANDOMIZE

Randomization can be performed by using mechanical methods, such as tossing a coin or rolling a die. These methods are time consuming, cumbersome, and not documented (i.e., cannot subsequently be checked). Using a table of random numbers (as in Table 8.1) is a generally preferred technique. In this table, the digits 0 to 9 are arranged in random order. By proceeding along one or more adjacent rows (or up or down one or more adjacent columns) of digits, it is possible to randomly allocate the treatments to the patients. The objective is to translate the sequence of random numbers into a sequence of randomized treatment assignments which can be used to implement the randomization of treatments to the patients entering the trial. The manner of executing the randomization varies according to the nature and requirements of the trial. I shall discuss only the most common procedures.

Known Sample Size

Consider, first of all, that the total sample size (or sample size within a stratum) is specified to be N before the start of the trial. The procedure is as follows. The numbers 1 through N are assigned to the patients to enter the trial. A random starting point in the random numbers table is selected, and proceeding along the rows (or down the columns), the numbers 1 to N are recorded in the order in which they occur (ignoring repetitions and numbers greater than N) to obtain a random permutation (variation in the order) of N. Finally, the random permutation of N is divided from left to right into groups of the

TABLE 8.1 Random Numbers

	0-9	10-19	20-29	30-39	40-49
0-4	23 01 71 61 37	30 99 22 70 87	30 99 22 70 87	90 76 31 69 17	66 50 09 39 49
	31 96 19 68 07	01 08 54 20 73	01 08 54 20 73	70 16 32 99 69	60 26 04 43 61
	11 13 63 24 47	09 74 65 74 23	09 74 65 74 23	67 62 23 74 57	88 45 75 23 37
	01 04 41 35 27	64 93 32 15 29	64 93 32 15 29	44 48 76 58 68	42 03 95 62 67
	81 97 31 17 89	79 01 62 98 46	79 01 62 98 46	95 31 96 60 18	04 23 06 30 27
5-9	50 73 06 39 73	31 17 08 73 17	82 25 28 53 13	13 89 23 88 30	63 58 27 96 73
	45 80 89 69 92	55 94 22 18 82	40 01 78 50 05	99 69 41 08 09	37 55 01 61 59
	71 82 70 81 33	98 20 37 98 58	32 45 29 17 82	34 69 12 10 65	48 98 02 70 73
	22 02 66 22 47	74 13 55 59 05	59 17 16 04 51	51 39 51 55 05	68 88 09 80 01
	68 45 81 50 20	76 25 27 76 48	69 12 97 38 36	05 07 18 99 83	57 03 21 00 04
10-14	03 03 51 04 64	13 96 43 74 57	46 78 08 83 74	01 69 74 69 21	80 15 88 25 76
	50 70 60 26 87	81 22 51 33 44	91 84 81 45 03	26 87 94 08 38	21 32 43 02 37
	57 00 77 75 33	99 53 56 05 34	51 67 04 69 88	28 42 29 46 50	69 41 29 86 14
	90 51 71 24 69	45 32 39 84 51	65 12 14 15 85	34 52 03 81 54	30 33 02 87 68
	75 75 65 95 33	23 72 86 82 80	33 86 45 62 13	19 39 82 43 20	14 06 77 39 33
15-20	75 98 56 87 90	71 01 76 65 72	95 50 69 19 43	31 97 79 48 40	04 29 97 46 03
	19 43 10 64 11	67 75 19 59 29	46 46 26 90 30	11 24 91 13 98	50 02 32 24 48
	86 33 76 92 25	44 37 06 75 56	48 74 43 29 22	32 92 85 43 29	19 33 57 28 58
	12 07 95 04 75	60 11 36 64 61	36 33 29 39 22	43 21 04 30 14	23 52 06 74 24
	75 06 09 85 74	57 96 27 48 51	63 43 33 83 04	10 53 89 14 98	62 91 46 48 76

A(19,2)   C(7,21)   B(12,47)

Source: Ref. 8.

appropriate size; there should be the same number of groups as treatments. The numbers contained in each group correspond to those patients who will receive a specified treatment, and from these the randomized treatment sequence can be generated.

For example, suppose that two treatments are to be allocated to 10 patients such that there are 5 patients in each treatment group, and the random starting point is point A in Table 8.1. Proceeding from left to right, treating a 0 as a 10, and ignoring repetitions of the same number, the random permutation is 7 4 9 5 0 6 1 3 2 8. The first five numbers in the random permutation of 10 (i.e. 7 4 9 5 0) correspond to those patients who receive one treatment, while the second five numbers in the random permutation of 10 (i.e., the remaining numbers 6 1 3 2 8) correspond to those patients who receive the other treatment. Note that we could have stopped after obtaining only the first five numbers, since the remaining numbers would automatically be assigned to the other group. Also, if $10 < N \leq 100$ the random numbers would be taken two at a time, 00 meaning 100, and so on.

Unknown Sample Size

Now suppose that the sample size is unknown. In this situation, some thought should be given to whether equality of numbers in the different treatment groups is required. If it is not necessary to have equal numbers in the groups, the procedure is as follows. The patients are to be entered serially, assigning to each patient in turn the number obtained by following a random sequence of digits in the random numbers table. Each patient is allocated to the treatment group determined by the interpretation of his or her number. This interpretation depends on the number of treatment groups.

For example, for equal probability allocation of two treatments (a and b, say), the patient receives a if the random number is odd, and b if the number is even. For equal probability allocation of three treatments (a, b, and c, say), the patient receives a if the number is 1, 2, or 3, b if the number is 4, 5, or 6, or c if the number is 7, 8, or 9 (zeros are ignored). For such a three-treatment trial, entering Table 8.1 at point B produces the sequence of treatments b a b c b a c a a b, corresponding to the random numbers 6 1 4 9 5 1 7 1 2 4.

Generally, however, it is advantageous to have equal numbers of patients in the treatment groups. If the sample size N is initially unknown, this may be achieved by <u>balanced block randomization</u> which ensures that the numbers in the different treatment groups are equal after every successive block of randomizations. A block size m (e.g., 4, 10, or 20) is specified, and to every block of m patients, the technique described for random allocation is applied where the sample size is m instead of N. For example, if m = 6 and there are two treatments, then in each successive block of six patients, one treatment is randomly allocated to three patients and the other treatment is allocated to the remaining three patients. Balance is achieved after every 6, 12, 18, and so on, patients. The numbers in the treatment groups are exactly balanced after every m patients, and are approximately balanced after the total intake of N patients if N is not a multiple of m. For example, Table 8.1 is entered at point C and only values in the range 1 to 6 are used. Reading across rows, the first three numbers are 2, 3, and 4, which defines the first block of six assignments, i.e., the sequence b a a a b b for the two treatments a and b. Likewise, the next three random numbers 5, 2, and 1 define the next block of six assignments, and so on.

Refinements and extensions to the randomization procedures described are endless; a review of the various procedures is given by Simon (2). In the final appraisal it is the individual who must judge, in the light of the particular study, the method of randomization to be employed and the benefits to be subsequently incurred.

8.3 DISCUSSION
Selection Bias

<u>Lachin</u>
One thing desired through randomization is to prevent the physician being able to break the code. If the physician knows that every sixth treatment is going to be such that there is an equal balance between a and b, and if he knows the first five assignments, then he will know what the sixth one will be. If the study is double blinded, however, he

cannot know. Thus, I generally do not recommend balancing within blocks unless a double-blind procedure is to be employed. Even then one might take added precautions, such as variable length blocks. Otherwise it is very easy for the physician to allow patient characteristics to influence the treatment allocation.

Chalmers

I think this is probably the most important point of randomization, that the doctor not be able to destroy the comparability of the treatment groups by altering the types of patients who get into each study group. To understand this I think we have to appreciate that not every patient who goes to a physician participating in a study is admitted to that study. A good protocol has a precise description of the kind of patient that will be admitted and the kind of patient that will be rejected, but within these definitions there are always leeways for subjective impressions, leeways for bias. One doctor will admit a patient whom another would not. If we acknowledge that two physicians would do it differently, we then have to acknowledge that if a doctor knows which treatment is coming next, he may be inclined to admit a patient whom he thinks might do well on that treatment, or he might be inclined to reject a patient whom he thinks might do badly on that treatment. In other words, we do not have true randomization if the physician has any suspicion of which treatment is coming next and is then able to restrict which types of patients enter each group. This can introduce a devastating bias since quite often only about 10% of the eligible patients are randomized into a study for various reasons.

Informed Consent

Let me illustrate how this can happen. We have not yet discussed informed consent, which is necessary for a patient to enter a study. The study must be explained to the patient and the patient must give consent. Ordinarily we think that a patient turns down the study because of stubbornness, or lack of interest, or disagreeing with the study. But the real reason a patient turns us down quite often is that we want him to turn us down. When a surgeon who is enthusiastic about an operation approaches a patient, he always gets that patient's permission to perform the operation. When a surgeon has doubts, or when an intern has doubts about the operation being good for that particular patient, he asks the patient's permission in such a way (unconsciously perhaps) that the patient refuses to give his permission. If randomization has broken down and the doctor knows which treatment is coming next, and it happens to be the treatment that is better or worse in his mind, then he has a great deal of influence on the assignment of patients in that study.

Why Randomization Is Essential; How to Do It   113

This is why I think that a number of randomized studies that seem to be well done turn out to have opposite conclusions. Although they are called randomized and controlled they are not done with absolute blinding, and patients become loaded in one group or the other as if the doctors were outwardly assigning the patients.

Implementing Randomization

It was said that flipping a coin was acceptable but awkward. I disagree, because flipping a coin does not provide a preassigned list of which treatment is to be assigned to each incoming patient, and it does not allow later checking to be sure that each patient enrolled into the study received the treatment intended as assigned by the randomization. A physician's bias may be so strong that he can flip a coin and it comes down heads, but he looks at it and there it is: tails. The patient then gets the treatment called for by tails when in fact the other less favorable treatment was assigned.

On the other hand, suppose the physician is given an envelope labeled for patient 42 on the outside, and it is a brown envelope, so he can't hold it up to the light and peek. If the physician then writes the name of the patient on the envelope and on the paper inside which says that patient 42 shall have treatment a, then there is a record that no mistake was made. The physician may still go ahead and start the other therapy because his bias is so strong that he does not realize he is cheating. Controls against bias should be built in at every step, and therefore flipping a coin is totally unacceptable.

Lachin

Whatever procedure for randomization is used, it is important that the entire randomization sequence, the entire randomization list, be generated before the start of the study. The randomization should then be inspected and some judgment exercised as to what is acceptable and what is not. It should be studied very carefully.

It has been shown, for example, that when a physician starts a clinical study he has a reservoir of good patients he knows he can tap in the beginning of the study. He will get these patients into the study and then he will have to start looking for other patients. These later patients may still meet all the criteria for entry, but their prognoses may not be as good and they will be different in many respects from the first group of patients to come into the study. Thus, it should be assured that the first 10 or 20 patients to be entered would not all be randomized into group a. Such a randomization sequence might be very rare, but if it arose, the sensible thing in my opinion is to do another randomization, and perhaps another, until an acceptable randomization sequence is generated, considering factors such as the early patients being different from the later patients.

Based on this concept, a number of computerized randomization procedures have been developed to apply what is called <u>constrained randomization</u> (3-5). In effect, these procedures place limits at each stage of the randomization process on the imbalance between group a and group b which is acceptable. Steps then are taken to ensure that at any stage in the sequence, an imbalance does not occur.

<u>Schoenfield</u>
One might ask why not just use the sequence a b a b a b whereby the first patient is assigned treatment a, the next patient treatment b, and so on. We have been talking about the disadvantage of such systematic sequences from the point of view of the doctor's bias, but there is another reason this is bad. Such systematic sequences are then subject to systematic error. If, for example, it was decided that patients coming into the Monday clinic will receive treatment a, and those coming into the Thursday clinic will receive treatment b, it may turn out that the patients that come on Monday come from one part of the town with a certain set of characteristics and the patients that come on Thursday come from another part with another set of characteristics. It may then happen that these characteristics will influence the results of treatment.

Blinding

<u>Lachin</u>
Another important consideration is the establishment of the double blind. Blinding can be implemented on a group or individual patient level. On the group level, a system such as the envelope system described above is used to assign treatment a or b to each patient. Andre Blum already described such a study in Chapter 4. The physician, however, then knows all the patients in the a group and all those in the b group. It is then very easy for the study to be biased if the physician is able to guess which treatment is which, and even though he may not be able to, at least subconsciously he can't keep from trying. Another problem is that if any one patient is unblinded (often patients will actually have their capsules analyzed), then all the patients in that group are unblinded, and the whole study is unblinded.

On the individual patient level, however, the treatment assigned to one patient is in no way linked to that assigned to other patients, and unblinding any one patient does not destroy the whole blind. For example, individual patient blinding would be achieved by having a separate patient supply of medication for each patient, such as bottles labeled for patients 1, 2, and so on. Rather than having an envelope for patient 42 saying a or b, the physician would have a bottle of capsules for patient 42 where only the biostatistician who generated the randomization and the drug supplier who bottled the pills know the contents, not the patient or physician or pharmacist. Such a mechanism has been employed in many studies and is described in detail in Ref. 6 or 7.

REFERENCES

1. Blumgart, H. T., Caring for the patient. N. Eng. J. Med., 1964, 270, 449-456.
2. Simon, R. H., Adaptive treatment assignment methods and clinical trials. Biometrics, 1977, 33, 743-749.
3. Efron, B., Forcing a sequential experiment to be balanced. Biometrika, 1971, 58, 403-417.
4. Pocock, S. J., and Simon, R., Sequential treatment assignment with balancing for prognostic factors in the controlled clinical trial. Biometrics, 1975, 31, 103-115.
5. Shaw, L. W., Ellenberg, S. S., Lachin, J. M., and Schlesselman, S. E., Constraints employed in randomization procedures, Proceedings of the Fifth Annual Symposium on Coordinating Clinical Trials, Arlington, Va., May 25-26, 1978, National Technical Information Service, No. PB 289-461.
6. Coronary Drug Project Research Group, The Coronary Drug Project: Design, methods and baseline results. Circulation, 1973, 47, 11-150.
7. Lachin, J. M., Marks, J. W., Schoenfield, L. J., and the NCGS Protocol Committee, and the National Cooperative Gallstone Study Group, Design and methodological considerations in the National Cooperative Gallstone Study: A multicenter clinical trial. Controlled Clinical Trials, 1981, 2, 177-230.
8. Petrie, A., Lecture Notes on Medical Statistics, Blackwell, London, 1978.

ADDITIONAL READINGS

Byar, D. P., Simon, R. M., Friedewald, W. T., Schlesselman, J. J., DeMets, D. L., Ellenberg, J. H., Gail, M. H., and Ware, J. H., Randomized clinical trials--perspectives on some recent ideas. N. Engl. J. Med., 1976, 295, 74-80.

Gehan, E. A., and Freireich, E. J., Nonrandomized controls in cancer clinical trials. N. Engl. J. Med., 1974, 290, 198-203.

Green, S. B. and Byar, D. P., The effect of stratified randomization on size and power of statistical tests in clinical trials. J. Chron. Dis., 1978, 31, 445-454.

Mantel, N., Random numbers and experimental design. American Statistician, 1969, 23, 32-34.

The Rand Corporation, A million Random Digits With 100,000 Normal Deviates, The Free Press of Glencoe, New York, 1955.

Weinstein, M. D., Allocation of subjects in medical experiments. N. Engl. J. Med., 1974, 291, 1278-1306.

Zelen, M., The randomization and stratification of patients to clinical trials. J. Chron. Dis., 1974, 27, 365-374.

9
Statistical Inference in Clinical Trials

JOHN M. LACHIN
The George Washington University
Washington, D.C.

9.1 INTRODUCTION TO INFERENCE

The aim of any clinical trial is to allow one to reach a conclusion, or in statistical terms an inference, as to the relative merits of a therapy in the face of variation. To quote the scientist-philosopher Jacob Bronowski (1), "All information is imperfect. We have to treat it with humility. That is the human condition. . . . Errors are inextricably bound up with the nature of human knowledge. . . ." All inferences, therefore, are to some degree uncertain and the statistical language of uncertainty is probability.

Statistical inference can be viewed as a simple decision problem, true or false, go or no-go. The principles of statistical inference are based on a consideration of the errors which might be made in making any decision about the truth or falsehood of a statement. In this case, the decision is based wholly on the results of a statistical test, and the decision problem can be expressed as in Table 9.1.

The process of statistical inference starts with a statement called the <u>null hypothesis</u> H_0, which specifies, for example, that the two therapies under consideration are not different, i.e., there is no real

TABLE 9.1 Types of Error in Statistical Inference

Statistical test result	Hypothesis	
	H_0 true	H_0 false
Significant (Reject H_0)	False positive (α)	True positive ($1 - \beta$)
Not significant (Fail to reject H_0)	True negative ($1 - \alpha$)	False negative (β)

difference between the two sample groups apart from that which might occur under random variation. Based on the observed measurements or set of data, a statistical test is then conducted and its results examined. The test results are usually expressed as a p-value which is simply the probability of obtaining a sample difference that is as great as or greater than that observed if in fact H_0 is true. If this p-value is less than some small a priori specified amount α, say 0.05 or 0.01, the hypothesis H_0 is then rejected because the probability of observing this set of data if H_0 were true is at least as small as α.

One type of error which then can occur is that the null hypothesis H_0 is rejected when it is really true. In this case, a false positive result is obtained and an error of type I is committed. The probability of this type I error is called the significance level, or just α. This event is the upper left cell of the above 2 x 2 table. Note that the probability α is in fact a conditional probability; α is the probability of a false positive result given that H_0 is true. Thus, the probabilities sum to unity (1.0) under H_0 true and also under H_0 false.

In formulating the decision problem, rather than merely stating that H_0 is false, one could be more precise and state that an alternative hypothesis H_1 is true. In a clinical trial, H_1 is the statement of the a priori specified minimal amount by which it is desired that the two therapies should in fact differ, namely, the minimal, clinically relevant difference as described in Chapter 4.

Now suppose that H_1 is true, but the statistical test result does not reach statistical significance; that is, the trial fails to reject H_0 when in fact H_0 is false. In this case a false negative result is obtained and an error of type II is committed. The probability of this type II error is β. If H_1 is true, however, and the statistical test result does reach statistical significance, then a true positive result is obtained. The probability of this occurring is called the power of the experiment, or just $1 - \beta$.

Thus, two types of error can occur: a false positive result with probability α and a false negative result with probability β. This is analogous to the problem of evaluating a diagnostic test result, as shown in Table 9.2. The objective is to determine from the diagnostic test whether a specific disease is absent or present, where the null hypothesis is that the disease is absent. The diagnostic test is conducted, and if the result is positive, the patient is inferred to have the disease. Otherwise, if the result is negative, the patient is inferred not to have the disease. Again the same two types of error may occur. The first is a false positive error, concluding that a patient has the disease because he displays a positive result, when in fact he is disease free. As before, its probability is α. The second is a false negative

TABLE 9.2 Types of Error in Diagnostic Decisions

Diagnostic test result	Disease	
	(H_0) Absent	(H_1) Present
Positive	(α) (False positive)	($1 - \beta$) (True positive)
Negative	($1 - \alpha$) (True negative)	(β) (False negative)

error, with probability β, in which it is concluded that the patient does not have the disease when in fact he does. As before, the power of the diagnostic test is the probability $1 - \beta$ of a true positive result, correctly saying that the patient has the disease.

In both these cases, statistical inference and the diagnostic test, the problem is formulated in terms of a <u>decision rule</u> and the types of error which might result from the long-run application of that rule under the competing conditions--H_0 true or H_1 true. We now consider how these concepts apply in conducting a standard statistical test.

9.2 THE STATISTICAL TEST

All commonly used statistical tests (t-test, chi-square, etc.) are based on the principle depicted graphically in Figure 9.1. One starts by defining a <u>test statistic</u> T which is to be applied to the observations, such as a t-test or a chi-square test, and which in some way reflects the observed difference between treatment and control. Figure 9.1 displays a test statistic T which is normally distributed with a mean value μ and a known variance Σ^2, which in turn is a known function of the variance σ^2 of the individual measurements. A null hypotheses H_0 is then specified about the true parameter of interest, e.g., the true mean or the true proportion of successes. In Figure 9.1, the mean of T is hypothesized to be μ_0 under H_0, where μ_0 is usually zero, and the probability distribution of T when H_0 is true is displayed.

A <u>critical region of size α</u> is then defined such that the probability of T falling in this region is some small quantity α when H_0 is true. In Figure 9.1 this region is defined as all values of T greater than a <u>critical value</u> T_α, where the corresponding area under the curve for H_0 is of size α. The statistic T is then calculated from the obtained sample of measurements, and if the value of T falls in the critical region, H_0 is rejected on the grounds that the probability of such an event is small if H_0 really were true; i.e., the result is <u>statistically significant</u>. Thus, if H_0 is true, the probability of a false positive result (type I error) is fixed at the a priori specified significance level α.

Statistical Inference   121

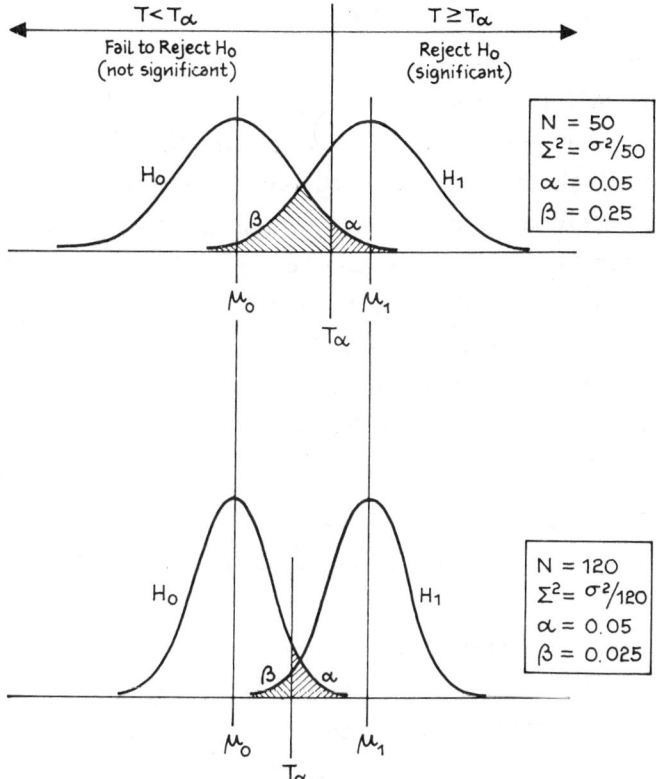

FIGURE 9.1 Rejection of the null hypothesis H_0 and the probabilities of type I (false positive) error α and type II (false negative) error β. The lower curve displays the effects on β when the sample size N is increased.

To conduct the test of significance, however, it is not necessary to specify the alternative hypothesis μ_1 or compute the power of the test $1 - \beta$ since the procedure assures that the type I error will not exceed α by the nature of the critical value T_α. Also, the critical region of size α is constructed such that the test will be assured of having maximum power (minimum β) in reference to the alternative H_1, although "maximum" only means that power is as large as it can be made to be, not that it is acceptably large.

To determine the actual power of the experiment, however, an alternative hypothesis must be specified about the parameter of interest. In Figure 9.1, the alternative hypothesis specifies that the mean of T is actually the value μ_1 where μ_1 is greater than μ_0. In this case μ_1 is the minimal, clinically relevant difference which one hopes to detect if in fact a difference of this magnitude exists. The probability distribution of T when H_1 is true then can be used to determine the power $1 - \beta$ of the study as displayed in the figure. If the test result does not fall in the critical region of size α, the trial fails to reject H_0; but if H_1 is true, this is a false negative result. The probability of this result, therefore, depends on a number of factors.

From an examination of Figure 9.1, the following relationships now can be seen to apply.

1. As α decreases, β increases and power $1 - \beta$ decreases, other factors constant.
2. As μ_1 increases, β decreases (power increases).
3. As variance Σ^2 decreases, β decreases (power increases).
4. As sample size N increases, β decreases (power increases).

Obviously, item 1 results by shifting the critical value T_α to the right, thus decreasing α. The obvious corollary is that as α is increased by shifting T_α to the left, then β decreases and power increases.

In item 2, the minimal, clinically relevant difference μ_1 becomes a critical specification in considering power once α has been fixed. In testing the difference between two alternate therapies in a clinical trial, μ_1 is usually specified as that difference between the two therapies which would lead one therapy to be preferred over the other, all factors being considered, such as the severity of the disease and the cost of the therapy. Obviously, the power of a study is highly dependent on the specification of μ_1. If μ_1 is increased, the entire curve for H_1 is shifted away from μ_0, thus decreasing β. The converse applies if μ_1 is decreased.

9.3 THE IMPORTANCE OF SAMPLE SIZE

Now we come to Σ^2, N, and β. The basis for item 3 above is that the variance of the test statistic determines the "spread" of the distribution of T under H_0 and H_1. The greater the variance, the wider the spread and the greater will be β. Thus, β can be reduced by selecting a more homogeneous sample for study in order to reduce Σ^2. One can, however, have a greater effect on the variance of the test statistic by adjusting the sample size. This is the basis for item 4 and is also illustrated in Figure 9.1. The basic relationship is that if the individual observations have variance σ^2, then the variance of the sample mean based on N observations becomes $\Sigma^2 = \sigma^2/N$.

In the upper part of Figure 9.1, for the μ_0 and μ_1 specified, a sample size of 50 was used to calculate T, α is 0.05, and β is 0.25. In the lower part of the figure are displayed the effects of increasing the sample size by a factor of 2.4 to N = 120; α is 0.05 as before, but now β is 0.025. (Note that by changing the sample size, the critical value for the test statistic is also changed to reflect the change in its variance.) Thus, it is through the variance of the test statistic that sample size becomes a dominant factor. The objective of sample size determination, therefore, is to select a sample size so that the clinical trial will achieve the desired value for β, and the desired level of power $1 - \beta$.

This clearly emphasizes the importance of sample size determination and the evaluation of power. It is never certain that the results of a clinical trial will reach significance if H_0 is false. If the test statistic does reach significance, the meaning is very clear; the probability of a false positive result is limited to the significance level α. In cases in which the test fails to reach significance, however, the power of the test becomes a critical factor in reaching an inference. Often, failure to achieve significance may be related more to the low power of the study (small sample size) than to an actual lack of difference between the competing therapies. Studies with inadequate sample size are thus doomed to failure before they begin and serve only to confuse the issue of determining the most effective therapy for a given condition. This is a critical issue in clinical research.

Conversely, in a study in which the power of detecting a specified clinically relevant difference μ_1 is sufficiently high, say 0.95, failure to achieve significance may properly be interpreted as probably indicating negligible relevant difference between the competing therapies. Thus, the proper interpretation of a negative result is based wholly upon a consideration of the power of the study. These considerations were illustrated by Freiman et al. (2) who showed that of 71 recent clinical trials which reached a negative result, 67 had power less than 0.90 in detecting a moderate (25%) therapeutic improvement. Their conclusion is that many of the therapies studied were not given a fair test simply due to inadequate sample sizes and thus inadequate power.

9.4 EVALUATION OF SAMPLE SIZE AND POWER

For each method of statistical analysis, there is a precise mechanism for determining sample size and power (3). For some statistical procedures this process is complex, but for most a simple approximate procedure exists (4). Through these methods, the adequacy of the sample size and the level of power can be evaluated when planning or analyzing the results of a study.

There are basically three types of questions which could be asked in the evaluation of sample size or power:

1. What total <u>sample size</u> N is required to ensure power $1 - \beta$ of detecting a clinically relevant difference μ_1?
2. What is the <u>power</u> $1 - \beta$ of the experiment in detecting a clinically relevant difference μ_1 when a specific sample size N is employed?
3. What <u>difference</u> μ_1 can be detected with power $1 - \beta$ if the experiment is conducted with a specified sample size N?

Question (1) usually is employed in planning a trial, and question (2) usually is employed in evaluating the results of a trial. Question (3) can be employed in either case.

Lachin (4) has shown that for a variety of statistical procedures most commonly employed in clinical trials, sample size N or power can be evaluated through the simple equations

(1) $$N = \left(\frac{Z_\alpha + Z_\beta}{K}\right)^2$$

or

(2) $$Z_\beta = K\sqrt{N} - Z_\alpha$$

In these equations, the terms Z_α and Z_β are constants affiliated with the desired α and β levels. These are simply the corresponding normal deviates such as

α or β	Z_α one-tailed	Z_α two-tailed	Z_β
0.01	2.327	2.575	2.327
0.05	1.645	1.960	1.645
0.10	1.281	1.645	1.281
0.20	0.841	1.281	0.841

In solving for power, one solves for Z_β and then uses a table of the normal distribution to find β (and then $1 - \beta$). For values of $Z_\beta < 0$, power will be < 0.50

To use these simple equations, the value K represents the measure of the clinically relevant difference to be detected (Δ) relative to the standard deviation of the observations (σ). Thus, K is of the general form $K = \Delta/\sigma$. For t-tests, tests for proportions, survival analysis, and tests for correlations, Lachin (4) presents the expressions for K and gives the precise sample size equations when this simplification is not possible. Using these methods, Lachin (5) has reviewed the sample size considerations for phase I, II, and III trials of investigational new drugs.

TABLE 9.3 Total Sample Size N from Eq. (1) as a Function of K for Various α (one-sided) and β

K	$\alpha = 0.05$ $\beta = 0.20$	$\alpha = 0.05$ $\beta = 0.10$	$\alpha = 0.01$ $\beta = 0.05$
0.025	9,898	13,708	25,232
0.05	2,476	3,428	6,308
0.075	1,100	1,524	2,804
0.10	620	858	1,578
0.15	276	382	702
0.20	156	216	396
0.25	100	138	254
0.3	70	96	176
0.5	26	36	64

Source: Ref. 4.

TABLE 9.4 Power $1 - \beta$ from Eq. (2) as a Function of K and Total Sample Size N with $\alpha = 0.05$ (one-sided).

N	K						
	0.05	0.10	0.15	0.20	0.25	0.30	0.50
20	0.0776	0.1155	0.1650	0.2265	0.2991	0.3808	0.7228
50	0.0983	0.1741	0.2795	0.4087	0.5489	0.6831	0.9707
100	0.1261	0.2595	0.4424	0.6387	0.8037	0.9123	0.9996
300	0.2180	0.5347	0.8297	0.9656	0.9964	0.9998	0.9999
500	0.2991	0.7228	0.9563	0.9977	0.9999	0.9999	0.9999
750	0.3914	0.8629	0.9931	0.9999	0.9999	0.9999	0.9999
1000	0.4745	0.9354	0.9990	0.9999	0.9999	0.9999	0.9999

Source: Ref. 4.

From Eq. (1), Table 9.3 presents total sample size N as a function of K, α, and β; while from Eq. (2), Table 9.4 presents power (from Z_β) as a function of K and N for $\alpha = 0.05$ (one-sided). Table 9.5 presents the expression for K for the more common statistical tests used in clinical trials assuming equal sample sizes. Lachin (4) presents the corresponding expressions for K in the case of unequal sample sizes and for other experimental designs not presented here.

The t-test

For the t-test of the equality of group means, Table 9.5 presents the expression for K to be used with the basic two-independent-group design, as well as the cases in which there are correlated observations such as when the same individuals are measured at times a and b, and when there are two independent groups with paired observations (as before and after treatment). For the two-independent-group design, ν_c is the projected mean for the quantitative outcome measure in the control group, and ν_e that in the treated group which in turn corresponds to the minimal relevant difference $\mu_1 = \nu_e - \nu_c$ that is desirable to detect. It is assumed that the standard deviation of the measurements σ is equal in both populations.

In the evaluation of sample size or power for the t-test, a critical factor is the specification of σ. For the other cases to be considered (proportions and survival), the variances are not specified separately. Usually, a value for σ can be specified based on prior experiments using the same measurements, and in these cases it is best to use the largest value of σ expected. Often, a pilot study is helpful to provide an estimate of σ under the conditions to be used in the experiment to be conducted. Of course, if power is evaluated after an experiment was conducted with a given N, then the obtained estimate of the standard deviation should be employed.

Equations (1) and (2), however, will tend to overestimate power, and thus will tend to underestimate the required sample size, although this effect is increasingly negligible for increasing degrees of freedom

TABLE 9.5 Values K for Use with Tables 9.3 and 9.4 or Eqs. (1) and (2)

Statistical Test	μ_1 under H_1^a	K for equal sample sizes
1. t-tests for means[b]		
a. Two independent groups e and c	$\nu_e - \nu_c$	$\dfrac{\|\nu_e - \nu_c\|}{2\sigma}$
b. Paired observations, e.g., at times a and b	$\nu_b - \nu_a$	$\dfrac{\|\nu_b - \nu_a\|}{\sigma_d}$
c. Two independent groups with paired observations	$\delta_e - \delta_c$ $\delta_e = \nu_{eb} - \nu_{ea}$ $\delta_c = \nu_{cb} - \nu_{ca}$	$\dfrac{\|\delta_e - \delta_c\|}{2\sigma_d}$ or $\dfrac{\|\delta_e - \delta_c\|}{\sigma\sqrt{2(1-\rho)}}$ if $\sigma_a = \sigma_b = \sigma$
2. Tests for proportions		
a. Two independent groups e and c	$\pi_e - \pi_c$	$\tfrac{1}{2}\|\pi_e - \pi_c\|[\overline{\pi}(1-\overline{\pi})]^{-\tfrac{1}{2}}$ $\overline{\pi} = \tfrac{1}{2}(\pi_e + \pi_c)$

3. Survival analysis: exponential model

a. Two independent groups without censoring

$$\lambda_e - \lambda_c$$

$$\frac{|\lambda_e - \lambda_c|}{\lambda_e + \lambda_c}$$

b. Two independent groups with censoring at time t

$$\lambda_e - \lambda_c$$

$$|\lambda_e - \lambda_c|[2\phi(\lambda_e) + 2\phi(\lambda_c)]^{-\frac{1}{2}}$$

$$\phi(\lambda) = \lambda^2 \left(1 - \frac{1 - e^{-\lambda t}}{\lambda t}\right)^{-1}$$

c. Two independent groups with entry to time t_0 and censoring at time t

$$\lambda_e - \lambda_c$$

$$|\lambda_e - \lambda_c|[2\phi*(\lambda_e) + 2\phi*(\lambda_c)]^{-\frac{1}{2}}$$

$$\phi*(\lambda) = \lambda^2 \left(1 - \frac{e^{-\lambda(t-t_0)} - e^{-\lambda t}}{\lambda t_0}\right)^{-1}$$

[a] $\mu_0 = 0$ under H_0 for each statistical test.
[b] σ_d^2 = variance of observations; σ_d^2 = variance of differences $x_b - x_a$.
Source: Ref. 4.

(df) of the t-test. An adequate adjustment is obtained by the correction factor $f = (df + 3)/(df + 1)$, where fN patients should actually be employed after solving for N in Eq. (1), or alternately N/f used in Eq. (2) when solving for power. For the two-independent-group design, $df = N - 2$.

For example, consider a study in which a treated and control group are to be compared in their mean levels of a quantitative outcome measure such as serum cholesterol (milligrams per deciliter). Assume that σ is known not to exceed $\sigma = 100.0$ mg/dl and it is desirable to detect a difference $\mu_1 = (\nu_e - \nu_c) = 20.0$ mg/dl. From Table 9.5, $K = \mu_1/2\sigma = 0.10$. From Table 9.3 with $\alpha = 0.05$ (one-sided), $N = 858$ is required to ensure 90% chance of detecting this difference. This would yield a t-test on 856 df. Thus the correction factor is $f = 1.006$ and the final sample size desired is $fN = 860$ all total, or 430 per group.

Suppose, however, that the experiment was actually conducted with only 102 patients. The correction factor is 1.02, and thus Table 9.4 or Eq. (6) is employed with $N = 102/f = 100$. For $N = 100$ and $K = 0.10$, Table 9.4 shows that the experiment had about 26% power ($Z_\beta = -0.645$) of detecting a difference of $\mu_1 = 20.0$ mg/dl. If the experiment produced a negative result, however, Table 9.4 also shows that with $N = 100$, there was almost 100% power in detecting a difference for $K = 0.5$ or where $\mu_1 = 2K\sigma = 100.0$ mg/dl. Thus, one could safely rule out a difference on the order of $\mu_1 = 100.0$ mg/dl.

Proportions

For tests of proportions, the basic two-group design is presented; Lachin (4) also presents equations for use with correlated observations at times a and b, as well as for two-independent groups with paired observations.

For example, suppose a controlled clinical trial of a new therapy is being planned to compare the proportion of patients healed in a treated and a control group, in which the proportion of successes in the control group is not expected to be greater than $\pi_c = 0.05$. Further, the new therapy would be considered superior--cost, risks, and other factors considered--if $\pi_e = 0.15$, thus yielding $\mu_1 = (\pi_e - \pi_c) = 0.10$. Since $\bar{\pi} = \frac{1}{2}(\pi_e + \pi_c) = 0.10$ and $\bar{\pi}(1 - \bar{\pi}) = 0.09$, the expression for K in Table 9.5 yields K = 0.167. Using Eq. (1) with $\alpha = 0.05$ (one-sided) and $\beta = 0.10$ yields N = 310 (rounded up from 308.4) all total, or 155 patients per group.

Suppose, however, that the trial was conducted with only N = 100. Using Eq. (2) shows that the power of the experiment in detecting K = 0.167 is only 51%. If a negative result were obtained, however, we might wish to determine the power of having detected larger differences. From Table 9.4 we find that N = 100 yields 91.2% power for K = 0.30. Direct calculation then shows that for $\pi_c = 0.05$, $\pi_e = 0.275$, and $\mu_1 = 0.225$, the value for K = 0.305. Thus a true difference of this magnitude could confidently be ruled out.

Survival

Expressions for K are also presented in Table 9.5 for the comparison of survival in two groups assuming an exponential model. Under this model, the proportion of survivors at time t is given as $P_s(t) = e^{-\lambda t}$ with hazard rate λ. The hazard rate is also the reciprocal of the mean survival time (see Section 11.10). The first expression for K in Table 9.5 applies to studies in which all N patients are followed to the terminal event (death), i.e., until the last patient dies, and thus this provides the total number of events required. This plan, however, is usually impractical and the second case allows for censoring of patient recruitment and follow-up after t years. The third expression is more general and allows for entry of patients up to time t_0 (e.g., 3 years) in a study of t years duration (e.g., 5 years).

For example, consider that a clinical trial is conducted for a disease with moderate levels of mortality with hazard rate $\lambda_c = 0.30$, yielding 50% survivors after 2.3 years.* Suppose that treatment is

---

*Survival at 2.3 years is selected as a reference point along the survival curve. In this model, the complete t year survival curves are to be compared, not just at one point in time.

desired to yield a reduction in hazard to $\lambda_e = 0.2$, i.e., an increase in survival to 64% at 2.3 years. With equally sized groups, $\alpha = 0.05$ (one-sided) and $\beta = 0.10$, line 3a from Table 9.5 yields N = 216 without censoring, i.e., 216 patients all followed to time of death, 108 in each group. If the study was to be terminated after 5 years, and recruitment spanned the 5-year interval, then using line 3b yields N = 508 patients. Finally, if recruitment was to be terminated after the first 3 years of a 5-year study, then line 3c yields N = 378.

Note that under each plan, the sample size requirement is based on the need to accrue approximately 216 deaths during the study. Also note that if a fixed number of patients is to be studied, it is better for those patients to be recruited quickly and followed for a longer period of time than to extend the period of study and reduce the rate at which the patients enter the study.

9.5 INFERENCE FROM LIKELIHOODS

The presentation in Sections 9.1 through 9.4 describes the Neyman-Pearson system of statistical inference which is based on the desire to control the frequency of false positive and false negative errors. Often, this is termed the <u>frequentist</u> approach to statistical inference. This section introduces an alternate approach to statistical inference which is based on the concept of relative <u>likelihood</u>. In clinical trials there is an ethical need to continuously examine the accumulating data in order to stop the trial as soon as either therapy is proven to be superior or inferior (see Sections 7.5 and 7.6). The difference between these two approaches is readily demonstrated through their application to these interim analyses conducted during a clinical trial (see also Section 11.11).

In the conduct of interim analyses using a frequentist statistical test, such as the t-test, the repeated application of the test yields an increasingly higher probability of type I error after each test is conducted. For example, if the null hypothesis of no treatment-control difference is tested at the $\alpha = 0.05$ level (two-sided) after each block of n observations is obtained, then the overall realized probability of type I error increases with each successive test as follows (from Ref. 6).

Successive test	Accumulated sample size	Actual type I error (α)
1	n	0.05
2	2n	0.083
3	3n	0.107
4	4n	0.126
5	5n	0.142
.	.	.
10	10n	0.193

After the first n observations are obtained, the statistical test is conducted with "nominal" α level = 0.05. After 2n observations have been obtained and the second statistical test is conducted, an additional probability of 0.033 that the null hypothesis will be falsely rejected is accrued, yielding an overall type I error level of approximately 0.083. This overall type I error level then continues to increase with each successive test.

Likewise, if there are multiple dependent variables, then each successive statistical test using a different variable results in a higher overall probability of type I error than had been achieved previously. The result of multiple tests, therefore, is simply that once a statistical test is conducted at level α using a single sample of measurements, a significance test can never again be conducted with that same type I error level. The simple reality is that the Neyman-Pearson theory of statistical tests presented above assures type I error level α for only one statistical test on any one sample or portion thereof.

One solution to this problem would be to conduct each of the separate multiple tests of significance using a smaller "nominal" α level in order to realize the desired overall type I error level. For example, in the problem of sequential looks, if repeated tests of significance are conducted after each block of n observations is obtained, and if each test is conducted at nominal α = 0.0107, the realized type I error level overall will not exceed 0.05 after 10 such sequential tests (see Ref. 6). Similar adjustments can be made when multiple independent or dependent variables are employed (see Ref. 7).

The reason that this problem arises rests in the basic formulation of statistical testing employed. As an example, consider two distinct diagnostic tests (A and B) with different error probabilities as follows:

	A		B	
Test result	H_0 true (No disease)	H_1 true (Disease)	H_0 true (No disease)	H_1 true (Disease)
Positive (Reject H_0)	0.05 (α)	0.10	0.05 (α)	0.80
Negative	0.95	0.90 (β)	0.95	0.20 (β)

In each of these the probability of type I error is $\alpha = 0.05$, whereas the power of the two tests differs markedly. The basic system of statistical inference asks the question: How likely is one to have a positive result if one is truly absent of disease? For both diagnostic tests, this probability is 0.05.

The question asked by the physician, however, is: How likely is the patient to have the disease if the test result is positive? In this case, the quantity of interest is the ratio of the two relevant <u>likelihoods</u> of a positive result when the disease is either absent or present. For diagnostic test A this <u>likelihood ratio</u> 0.10/0.05 indicates that one is twice as likely to have the disease as to not have the disease if the test result is positive. For test B, however, the likelihood ratio 0.80/0.05 indicates that the patient is 16 times as likely to have the disease as to not have the disease if the diagnostic test result is positive. A similar interpretation may be applied to the comparison of two clinical trials with different sample sizes and thus different levels of statistical power.

This example points out that the significance level, $\alpha = 0.05$ in this case, alone is not an appropriate yardstick for the evaluation of statistical evidence. This simple example clearly disproves what has been referred to as the <u>alpha postulate</u>. The alpha postulate simply states that all null hypotheses rejected with significance level $\alpha = 0.05$ have equal evidence against them. This clearly is not so.

On the other hand, the likelihood ratio is a coherent and consistent measure of statistical evidence for or against an hypothesis. The reason obviously is that the likelihood ratio, as a measure of statistical evidence against the null hypothesis, is based on both α <u>and</u> power. The application of such methods to interim analyses in clinical trials is discussed in Section 11.11.

In summary, statistical inference requires that one make a judgment about the truth or falsity of a stated null hypothesis. Traditional procedures consider only the probability of the data that has been observed, assuming that the given null hypothesis being tested is true. Procedures based on likelihood ratios, however, are aimed at the question of how likely are the competing hypotheses in light of the data.

9.6 DISCUSSION
The Clinically Relevant Difference

<u>Ingelfinger</u>
I am confused by the reference to statistically significant differences on the one hand, and clinically relevant differences on the other. You have used the term clinically relevant difference quite often, but I don't think you mean it in the way Dr. Juhl used the term earlier (see Chapter 4).

<u>Lachin</u>
I definitely mean it that way, subjectively. The sample size is determined such that the study will have a good chance of detecting a difference that the physician considers to be clinically relevant. In my second example, a true difference of 10% between the treated group and the placebo group was considered clinically relevant by the investigators. Anything less was of no interest in treating their patients. If the study were not to have a high probability of producing a statistically significant result in light of a true clinically relevant

difference of 10%, then there is no point in doing the study. Would you be willing to embark on a study which only gave you a 30% chance (power) of finding a statistically significant difference when 10% was the true difference between the treated and control patients in the general population? That is the issue of sample size determination. The sample size is selected to give the study a high probability of achieving success statistically when the true difference between the groups is as great as that which the physician considers clinically relevant.

Schoenfield
Perhaps I can clarify by indicating how Dr. Lachin might have arrived at the figures in his example. He first would ask the clinicians in this particular study to estimate the spontaneous rate of occurrence of the desired effect, say treatment success, and the maximum figure might be only 5%. Then the next question to the clinicians would be to state the result the therapy should have for it to be considered clinically relevant. Suppose the answer is 15%, i.e., a 10% difference. Dr. Lachin would then have the information he needs to evaluate the sample size requirements as he did in his example.

Lachin
I tend to view my role as not specifying anything. The clinician specifies the difference he wishes to detect: the clinician specifies alpha, the clinician specifies beta. I simply use a formula to then evaluate the sample size. I do, however, help the clinician formulate an understanding of the problem, and reach a decision as to the objectives of the trial. Often this is an iterative process. The clinician first specifies what would be considered a clinically relevant difference, and from this the sample size required to yield a high probability of obtaining a significant result is determined. Sample size requirements might be examined for a range of clinically relevant effects or for various outcome measures before arriving at a final conclusion. To do this, however, it is important that the clinician understand that the degree of difference to be sought, the sample size to be used, and the type II error level (or power) are all interrelated.

Multiple Objectives

Ingelfinger
You indicated that trials often have multiple objectives, such as efficacy and safety. How is sample size evaluated in this case?

Lachin
The easiest way is to consider each objective separately, but even then this may not be a simple procedure. To detect toxicity you will always need many more patients than to detect efficacy. For a drug to be considered effective, a rather large difference is usually required (the clinically relevant difference). To evaluate safety, however, if a

suspected side effect is severe, a small difference is clinically relevant. Thus, it is not uncommon to discover that less than 100 patients per group are enough to detect efficacy but more than 2000 are required to detect small relevant rates of toxicity. Usually this is impossible, and one has to redefine the toxicity rates in terms of those differences in side effects which can likely be detected with a given sample size (question 3 in section 9.4). The final sample size is then determined considering cost, resources, and all of the objectives. In Reference 5 I have conducted a review of sample size considerations in the evaluation of potentially toxic drugs along these lines.

A good example of these various considerations is the sample size calculation for the National Cooperative Gallstone Study (NCGS) (8) which was described in the discussion in Chapter 4. For the assessment of efficacy, a 30% difference in dissolution rates was considered minimally, clinically relevant, requiring less than 100 patients per group. To detect a 1% difference in the rate of toxic effects, however, required over 1700 patients per group. This was clearly unreachable. We thus decided to consider the evaluation of efficacy among subgroups, such as among those with large versus small gallstones, and concluded that 300 patients per group would be adequate to detect a 15 to 20% differential between the subgroups in the degree of efficacy. With this as the sample size, it was then determined that the study would have a 95% chance (power) of detecting a 6 to 7% difference between the groups in the rates of toxic effects. This was considered to be an acceptable level of power for the evaluation of toxicity, and thus the final sample size was 300 patients in each group.

Tygstrup
I think that from the patient's point of view there is only one outcome: good or bad. The difficulty is that we cannot precisely balance risks and benefits.

Lachin
That balance is evaluated by doing the clinical trial, observing the risks and the benefits. A patient in the gallstone study may have all of his gallstones dissolved but end up with cirrhosis. This is a success in terms of efficacy but at the same time a failure in terms of toxicity. Thus, in reaching the final decision as to whether a therapy has a satisfactory risk-to-benefit ratio, all outcomes should be considered simultaneously.

Tygstrup
But the risk of toxicity from chenodeoxycholic acid also should be balanced against the risk of an attack of cholecystitis and then having the gallstones removed by surgery. If the risk of the treatment is to develop cirrhosis and the risk of having no treatment is to develop cholecystitis, you then have to consider how many cases of cholecystitis you will accept to avoid one case of cirrhosis.

Lachin
Analysis of the trial's results may help solve these problems. We hope to be able to show that patients with certain characteristics have a good chance for an effective therapy with no side effects, whereas other characteristics may indicate either a poor therapeutic prognosis or a high risk of complications.

The Importance of Sample Size

Chalmers
I have long been bothered by these issues. We have seen that only 1% of clinical trials in the literature are randomized controlled trials. How many of the authors of those 1% of randomized controlled trials understood the importance of adequate sample size? A clinical trial of prednisone in patients with acute alcoholic hepatitis found that prednisone was more effective than placebo at the $\alpha = 0.05$ level (9). It was considered a positive study, and physicians began to use prednisone to treat alcoholic hepatitis. Another article (10), appeared, however, which concluded that this treatment was not effective because a significant effect was not shown at the 5% significance level with their limited number of patients. Therefore, they recommended that the drug should not be used. The authors, however, did not understand how easy it was to miss a real effect with their small sample size (2). This is the crucial aspect of planning in a therapeutic trial, and this is why the biostatistician should be treated as a co-author from the beginning.

Implications For Publications

Ingelfinger
Dr. Chalmers has raised a practical question for you as authors and for me as an editor. Usually, an article does not state whether proper preliminary calculations have been carried out, and thus the practical question is whether every clinical trial published in a journal should have a paragraph in the methods section defining the minimal relevant clinical difference, α, β, and the calculation of the total number of patients necessary. As far as I know, the New England Journal of Medicine has received few papers with such introductions.

Lachin
I believe that much scientific reporting, including clinical trails, is deficient and that much of the analysis also may well be deficient since the usual statistical test does not consider the probability of false negative error β. Additional steps are necessary to do this, and such calculations are rarely reported.

Juhl
Among the 306 randomized clinical trials in the decade 1964-1973 on treatment in gastroenterology (see Chapter 3) only five trials mentioned the type II error β.

Ingelfinger

A related point is that papers are often full of statements that there was a difference or a trend, but the difference was not statistically significant. What is the poor reader or even the poor editor to interpret from such a statement? Sometimes I feel that if the authors have gone through the trouble to define whether it is significant, then why don't they just say, "there is no difference." Instead they qualify and say that there was not a statistically significant difference but there certainly was a strong trend.

Lachin

This is another general issue in all scientific reporting. Should the authors say that the difference is significant or not significant, and no more; or should they say it is not significant but there was a trend? The answer to that, in my opinion, depends on the reader. The reader who realizes that "not significant" means that significance just was not obtained in that particular study will not be confused. It may have been due to the fact the study had very poor power, meaning a small sample size, or it may be due to the fact that no difference really exists. This is why a negative statistical result by itself is insufficient ground to accept the null hypothesis as true. What is needed in this case is a statement of the power of the study to detect a relevant difference.

The reader needs all the information he can get. Data should be fully reported, but at the same time, the reader should not be misled, and this is the problem. When a physician reads a report in which it is zealously stated that the result was not significant but there was a trend, then he often thinks, "well, it is probably really there but he didn't get it." That is not the right attitude.

Riis

I want to be an advocate for the reader, if a significant difference is not found, then the risk of a type II error should be stated, and then please stop. The statement that there is a trend is really one's own belief and it should be left to the reader to form his own opinion. I think the innocent reader is misled by statements of "not significantly different, but there is a trend."

Lachin

Saying that there is trend is the problem. What is important is to point out that there was a difference, that it was not significant, and the level of power the study had to detect a specified clinically relevant difference.

Multiple Tests

Juhl

Dr. Lachin has mentioned the danger of multiple analyses of the data, and cautioned that only one look at the data is allowed with a usual simple significance test. I would like to show what could have happened if one had made repeated tests in a real trial. Figure 9.2 shows a trial

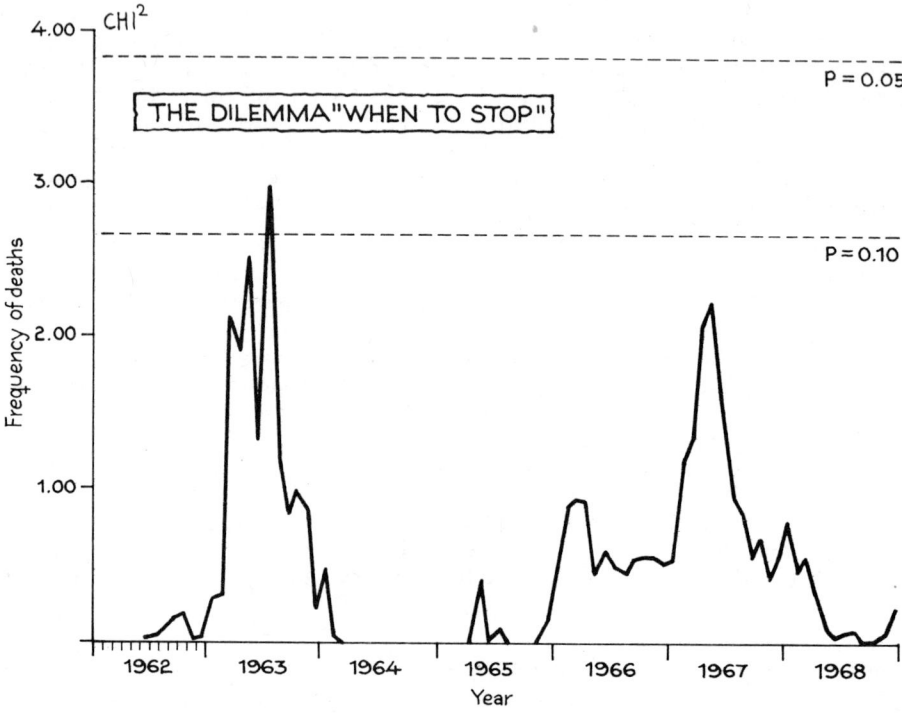

FIGURE 9.2 Chi-square tests performed retrospectively comparing the cumulative frequencies of deaths each month after the start of a controlled trial of prednisone in the treatment of 524 patients with cirrhosis (From Ref. 11).

which started in 1962 and ended in 1969 with no difference in survival between the treated and the control groups (11). During each year about 70 patients entered the trial, and retroactively we compared the cumulative death rate in the controls with that in the treated group using successive chi-square tests each month from the start of the trial. The chi-square value fluctuated greatly during the course of the trial, and if a type I error level of 10% had been chosen, we could have stopped the trial in 1963 with a positive result. At the end of the trial in 1969, however, we found no difference in survival. Here is the danger from a real example of making multiple looks and repeated testing of the accumulating data.

Lachin

As I pointed out, multiple looks are also a problem for subgroup analyses. There is a general rule that applies not only to repeated testing with more and more subjects, but also to examining more and more subgrouping variables. The more often the data are examined, the more likely something is to be found by chance alone.

Suppose a study is conducted and there are a number of variables which were measured because they might be related to the outcome of interest. There is then a big difference between the subgroup factors specified beforehand and those that just turn up in scrutiny of the data afterward. When a few subgroup factors are specified beforehand, rather simple steps such as using a smaller significance level can be used to adjust for the effects on type I error.

There is also a second general rule: a new hypothesis should never be tested with the data that lead to the generation of that hypothesis. Thus, it is very difficult, if not impossible, to evaluate or correct for the type I error when what is often called a fishing expedition is conducted, testing any number of subgroup factors just because they were available. For this reason I think it is acceptable to fish so long as post hoc subgroup results are reported as such when published so that others can conduct further trials to test the new hypotheses generated.

REFERENCES

1. Bronowski, J., The Ascent of Man, Little Brown and Co., Boston, Mass., 1973, pp. 353-360.

2. Freiman, J. A., Chalmers, T. C., Smith, H., and Kuebler, R., The importance of beta, the type II error and sample size in the design and interpretation of the randomized controlled trial. N. Engl. J. Med., 1978, 299, 690-694.

3. Cohen, J., Statistical Power Analysis for the Behavioral Sciences, Academic, New York, 1969.

4. Lachin, J .M., An introduction to sample size determination and power analysis for clinical trials. Controlled Clinical Trials, 1981, 2, 93-113.

5. Lachin, J. M., Sample size considerations for clinical trials of potentially hepatotoxic drugs, in Guidelines for Detection of Hepatotoxicity Due to Drugs and Chemicals (C. S. Davidson, C. M. Leevy, and E. C. Chamberlayne, eds.), U.S. Department of H.E.W., National Institutes of Health, NIH Publication No. 79-313, 1979, pp. 119-130.

6. McPherson, K., Statistics: The problem of examining accumulating data more than once. N. Engl. J. Med., 1974, 290, 501-502.

7. Kupper, L. L., Stewart, J. R., and Williams, K. A., A note on controlling significance levels in stepwise regression. Amer. J. of Epidemiol., 1976, 103, 13-15.
8. Lachin, J. M., Marks, J. W., Schoenfield, L. J., and the NCGS Protocol Committee, and the National Cooperative Gallstone Study Group, Design and methodological considerations in the National Cooperative Gallstone Study: A multicenter clinical trial. Controlled Clinical Trials, 1981, 2, 177-230.
9. Helman, R. A., Temko, M. H., Nye, S. W., and Fallon, H. J., Alcoholic hepatitis: Natural history and evaluation of prednisone therapy. Ann. Intern. Med., 1971, 74, 311-321.
10. Campra, J. L., Hamlin, E. M., Kirschbaum, R. J., Olivier, M., Redeker, A. G., and Reynolds, T. B., Prednisone therapy of acute alcoholic hepatitis: Report of a controlled trial. Ann. Intern. Med., 1973, 79, 625-631.
11. Tygstrup, N. and Juhl, E., Dilemmas of controlled clinical trials in hepatology, in The Liver and Its Diseases (F. Shaffner, S. Sherlock, and C. M. Leevy, eds.), Intercontinental Medical Book Corporation, New York, 1974, pp. 64-75.

ADDITIONAL READINGS

Canner, P. L., Monitoring treatment differences in long-term clinical trials. Biometrics, 1977, 33, 603-616.

Cornfield, J., Sequential trials, sequential analysis and the likelihood principle. American Statistician, 1966, 20, 18-23.

Cornfield, J., Recent methodological contributions to clinical trials. Am. J. Epidemiol., 1976, 104, 408-421.

Cutler, S. J., Greenhouse, S. W., Cornfield, J. and Schneiderman, M. A. The role of hypothesis testing in clinical trials. J. Chron. Dis., 1966, 19, 857-882.

Gibbons, J. D. and Pratt, J. W., p-Values: Interpretation and methodology. American Statistician, 1975, 29, 20-25.

Halperin, M., Rogot, E., Gurian, J. and Ederer, F., Sample sizes for medical trials with special reference to long-term therapy. J. Chron. Dis., 1968, 21, 13-24.

Lachin, J., Sample size determination for r x c comparative trials. Biometrics, 1977, 33, 315-324.

Meier, P., Statistics and medical experimentation. Biometrics, 1975, 31, 511-529.

Meier, P., Terminating a trial--the ethical problem. <u>Clin. Pharmacol. Ther.</u>, 1979, <u>25</u>, 633-640.

Wu, M., Fisher, M., and DeMets, D., Sample sizes for long-term medical trials with time-dependent dropout and event rates. <u>Controlled Clinical Trials</u>, 1980, <u>1</u>, 111-123.

10
Choice of Variables for Evaluation of Therapeutic Effect: The Statistical Point of View

AVIVA PETRIE*
London School of Hygiene and Tropical Medicine
and Royal Postgraduate Medical School
London, England

10.1 SCALES OF MEASUREMENT

The various components which constitute a clinical trial are inextricably linked such that a deficiency in any one of them has a substantial derogatory effect on the validity of the trial. Perhaps the most basic component to be considered is the selection of variables for evaluation of therapeutic effects.

It is clearly wise to commence by ensuring that the term variable, in the statistical context, is unambiguous and well defined. A variable is a characteristic which varies such that it may take any one of a specified set of values. A variable may be quantitatively or qualitatively measurable. If a variable is quantitative, such that each value may be expressed by a number, the variable may be subclassified as discrete or continuous. A discrete variable is one for which the number is obtained simply by counting, and such a variable has only a

---

*Ms. Petrie is currently with the London School of Hygiene and Tropical Medicine, London, England.

countable number of distinct possibilities. A <u>continuous</u> variable is one in which the number requires measurement such that there is no indivisible unit (e.g., the variable systolic blood pressure, which is measured in millimeters mercury). Alternately, a variable may be qualitative, in which case the "values" are coded numbers assigned to categories; either on a <u>nominal</u> (classificatory) scale defined by mutually exclusive unordered categories (e.g., blood groups AB, A, B, O), or on an <u>ordinal</u> or ranking scale defined by related categories (e.g., poor, average, good). Thus, variables may be characterized according to the <u>scale of measurement</u> on which they are defined. This typology involves the structure and meaning of the variables. The scale of measurement is important because it influences the methods of statistical analysis which may be employed.

Often the term parameter is substituted incorrectly for variable, and it is prudent here to clarify the distinction between variables, parameters, and statistics. A variable, as stated above, is a characteristic which varies. A <u>parameter</u> is a summary value which in some way describes the nature of the variable in the population under study. Often it is a mathematical function of the population values of the variable (e.g., the population mean, the population standard deviation). Generally, since not all the values of the variable in the population are known, the values of the parameters are unknown and they must be estimated. A <u>statistic</u> is also a summary value, but it is calculated from a sample of values of the variable, usually as an estimator of the (unknown) population parameter (e.g., the sample mean as an estimator of the population mean).

10.2 RESPONSE VERSUS CONCOMITANT VARIABLES

As a next stage, it is important to distinguish between dependent or response variables and prognostic or concomitant variables. The <u>response</u> variables are those variables which directly measure response to treatment. The <u>concomitant</u> variables are those which are thought to substantially influence response to treatment. Both the response and the concomitant variables play an important part in evaluating therapeutic effect as described in Chapters 5 and 6. It is to the former, whose role is perhaps the more marked, that discussion is now directed.

In all circumstances it is important to ensure that the chosen response variable is <u>relevant</u> to the aims of the trial, whether it be an assessment of therapeutic or adverse effects. Each may be equally important in judging the relative merits of treatments. Although seemingly obvious, it is all too easy to transgress from this directive, for example, by selecting those variables which are easily available.

The choice of the response variable is also dependent on the nature of the measurement. Response can be measured in <u>absolute</u> terms, the measurement on an individual comprising an observable quantitative value of the variable at the end of the treatment period (e.g., blood pressure in mmHg). These values for the patients in each group are then compared to evaluate treatment effect. Alternatively, response can be measured in <u>relative</u> terms, for example, the measurement being an indication of improvement of a condition over a period of time, such as the change of blood pressure from before to after treatment. In general, it is preferable that the response variable be measured in relative terms.

In addition, the timing of the measurements is also an important consideration and should also be relevant to the aims of the trial. A response variable, no matter how exact and appropriate, may still not be relevant if the timing of its measurement does not correspond with the timing of the anticipated effects.

10.3 RELIABILITY AND VALIDITY

The choice of variables may also be influenced by the reliability and validity of the response measure. These are statistical terms which have a precise meaning in the theory of tests and measurements as developed by psychometricians, but whose practical meaning is readily appreciated and assessed. <u>Reliability</u> refers to the degree to which the measurement varies on repeat testing, while <u>validity</u> refers to the degree to which the measurement approximates the true value of the variable for that individual.

For example, suppose that blood pressure is to be measured in a hypertensive patient and there are two different measuring instruments, say, instruments A and B. On a single patient, A gives two successive readings (diastolic) of 105 and 120 mmHg, while B gives 102 and 104 mmHg. Clearly instrument B is more reliable because it shows less variability on repeat testing. Suppose, however, that for this patient, at the time these readings were obtained, the <u>true</u> blood pressure was 114 mmHg. In this case instrument A appears to be more valid since "on the average" its values are closer to the true value than instrument B, the latter being more reliable but also showing a consistent tendency to underestimate blood pressure, at least in this patient.

Where possible, the reliability and validity of the response measurements should be assessed and described, especially where a novel measurement procedure is to be employed. There are many factors which enter into this assessment. An instrument's characteristics may be influenced by the degree of training of the observer or technician, the patient population under study, and the environment within which the observation is obtained. For example, the characteristics of instruments A and B might be highly different when used by a physician as opposed to a nurse assistant, or when used in a hypertensive as opposed to a normotensive population, when used with the patient standing, seated, or supine, before or after meals, morning or afternoon, and so on. Assessment of these characteristics is further discussed in Chapter 15.

10.4 OBJECTIVE VERSUS SUBJECTIVE MEASURES

The characteristics of reliability and validity are also related to the classification of response measures in terms of the varying degrees of objectivity versus subjectivity. Assessment of response may be purely objective, any deviation from the truth being a consequence only of recording or copying errors rather than observational error. The response "death" or "survival" is an example of an objective assessment of response. Alternatively, assessment of response may be semiobjective, the measurement (e.g., blood pressure using a standard sphygmomanometer) being subject to observational error reflected in the reliability and/or validity of the measurement. Various remedies have been suggested to remove or reduce these observational errors, for example, the installation of automatic recording facilities to remove observer variation, blind assessment (the observer being uninformed as to the treatment the patient is receiving), employing the same observer to assess response on all individuals, thus eliminating between-observer variation, and taking the average of repeat readings to reduce measurement variability (improve reliability).

Finally, assessment of response may be purely subjective, as in the case of the patient's own evaluation of his symptoms. The patient's assessment is subject to suggestion, and for this reason it is important to disassociate the "specific" or pharmacological effect of the treatment from the "nonspecific" or psychological effect of receiving treatment. There are various methods which achieve this separation and hence eliminate bias--most commonly, making the trial double blind, or using a placebo, or both. By its very nature, a subjective measure has lower reliability and validity than an objective or semiobjective measure.

A relevant subjective measure, however, should always be preferred to a nonrelevant objective measure. In Chapter 6, Dr. Blum made this point very clearly when he showed that gastric secretion in ulcer patients is a good objective measure, but may not be relevant to the outcome of interest, which is whether there is healing of the ulcer.

10.5 MULTIPLE VARIABLES

Discussion, thus far, has been limited to the choice of a single response variable. On a wider and more practical sphere, consideration should be given to the problem of coping with a multiplicity of response and/or concomitant variables. Let me begin, this time, with the latter.

In a clinical trial there are generally a number of concomitant or prognostic variables which are believed to influence response, and which should therefore in some way be taken into account in the statistical analysis, and possibly the design of the trial. The problem is to identify these variables and to decide how many warrant special attention, and what that attention, in statistical terms, should be. If too many concomitant variables are singled out, the repercussions are a desirability for an increasingly large number of patients, demands for endless subanalyses and recombinations, and thus a high probability that significant effects will be observed by chance alone. On the other hand, if the concomitant variables are totally ignored, biased analyses may result. Certainly this is a problem which is difficult to resolve. Randomization goes far to alleviate concern. In the case of a few particularly important concomitant variables which possibly require special study, stratified randomization may be an answer.

The problem of dealing with a multiplicity of response variables requires a different solution, for then it is the statistical analysis and the interpretation of results that are of prime importance. One simple approach is to perform a separate analysis for each response variable, but a difficulty may be encountered if these analyses produce conflicting results. Sometimes one response variable is considered to be of greatest consequence, and the conclusions based on the analysis of this variable can then take precedence. Another approach is to perform a multivariate analysis, considering all the variables in combination simultaneously. Although apparently the answer in principle, such analyses are not always feasible and can lead to reduced statistical power. In addition, they may not really seem to answer the questions raised.

Choice of Variables   151

10.6 IMPLICATIONS FOR ANALYSIS

Finally, once a decision has been reached as to which variables are to be chosen to evaluate therapeutic effects, some thought should be spared for the underlying assumptions of the proposed statistical analysis. The feasibility of many analyses is dependent on the assumptions of the analysis, and these may influence the manner in which the selected variables are handled. Different forms of analysis make different assumptions, and analyses may vary in their degree of robustness to violations of the assumptions, i.e., the degree to which they are insensitive to such violations. The assumption of a specific distributional form of the variable (of normality, in particular) is common, as are assumptions of linearity and of homogeneity of variance. These assumptions can often be validated by simple plots and inspection of the data. If these assumptions are violated, there are various courses of action to pursue, for example, the data may be transformed or nonparametric analyses may be performed. A nonparametric distribution-free test makes no assumptions about the distribution of the variable in the population being studied, while a parametric test does make some sort of assumption about the distribution of the data.

10.7 DISCUSSION

Types of Measurements

Lachin
It should be kept in mind that the different scales of measurements (quantitative versus qualitative) entail different forms of analysis which require different types of assumptions. No assumptions need be made about a variable that is of a nominal scale, such as male versus female or healed versus not healed. For such a nominally scaled variable, methods of analysis relevant to rates or proportions would be employed.

Another point is that if subjective measures are to be used, it is always advisable to to employ at least two observers. This way at least some information is obtained about the variability of the observations, and the observer bias. In a classic study, Yerushalmy (1) compared the independent evaluations of different radiologists in evaluating a series of x-rays. They were experienced radiologists, but they read the x-rays entirely differently. Had a study been done using just one observer there may not have been any question about the outcome observed, whereas a different observer might have lead to a different result. With two observers, there may perhaps be some confusion, but the study results should provide greater information.

Finally, it is always useful to collect concomitant variables that are auxiliary to those needed to evaluate the main objectives. I do not feel that one should only measure those variables that are absolutely essential to evaluate the trial's objectives. In science, more information can never be bad. The only real issue in collecting auxiliary information, apart from cost, is that it be properly handled.

Nonparametric Statistical Tests

Juhl
I would like to advocate more use of nonparametric distribution-free tests. They are simple to use, there are no requirements on the distribution of the data, and the efficiency is rather high in comparison to the parametric test.

Petrie
But they are not as powerful as the corresponding parametric test. If the assumptions of a parametric test are satisfied, such as the assumption of normality for the t-test, then this test will be more powerful than the analogous nonparametric test.

Juhl
But not very much so. If the population has a perfect normal distribution with equal variances in the two groups, and if 100 patients are needed to find a difference with a nonparametric test, the same difference can be found using only 95 patients if a t-test is used (2). This is the only loss if a nonparametric test is used, and I think it is a rather small one.

Lachin
A good example of a variable that usually violates the assumptions of a parametric test is age. Age is not going to have a distribution from $-\infty$ to $+\infty$. Ages below 0 are not possible, whereas a normal distribution assumes that there is a possibility of ages below 0. In addition, age may not be symmetrically distributed, i.e., may not have a bell shape. Thus, age may violate the assumption of normality which is required for the t-test.

A nonparametric test, however, makes no assumption about how age or any other variable is distributed; it makes no assumption about the shape of the frequency distribution. If a variable like age is to be analyzed, the only assumption is that it be a quantitative measurement. Each scale of measurement entails its own form of analysis, and there are nonparametric or distribution-free methods of analysis for quantitative variables, ordinal variables, and nominal variables (2). They are very easy to use, and as Dr. Juhl pointed out, their power for a given sample size is often 95 to 98% of what the power would be for the parametric test.

Chalmers
Nonparametric methods may offer a great amount of precision in detecting whether one drug is better than the other. The Crohn's Disease Study (3, 4) recognized that patients with Crohn's disease have all degrees of severity of illness, and it was desired to know whether a drug makes a sick patient better as well as keeps a well patient well. Therefore, a score system was constructed and a nonparametric method, the Wilcoxon rank order test, was used to get some information out of every patient (3). Every patient contributed a little bit to answering the question of the comparative efficacy of the drugs, because what were considered the good and the bad responses were rated beforehand.

For instance, death is the worst outcome, that patient is at the bottom of the list. A well patient is at the top of the list, and in between are hundreds of variables or degrees of changes which allowed all the patients to be ranked at the end of the study. By using this method it was thus possible to determine whether on the average the drug makes more people better than did the placebo (4).

REFERENCES

1. Yerushalmy, J., Statistical problems in assessing methods of medical diagnosis with special reference to x-ray techniques. Public Health Reports, 1947, 62, 1432-1439.

2. Siegel, S., Nonparametric Statistics for the Behavioral Sciences, McGraw-Hill, New York, 1956.

3. Best, R. B., Bectel, J. M., and Singleton, J. W., Rederived values of the eight coefficients of the Crohn's Disease activity index (CDA). Gastroenterology, 1979, 77, 843-846,

4. Summers, R. W., Switz, D. M., Sessions, J. T., Bectel, J. M., Best, W. R., Kern, F., and Singleton, J. W., National Cooperative Crohn's Disease Study: Results of drug treatment. Gastroenterology, 1979, 77, 847-869.

11
Statistical Analysis of the Randomized Clinical Trial

JOHN M. LACHIN
The George Washington University
Washington, D.C.

11.1 INTRODUCTION

This chapter reviews some of the basic issues and methods for the statistical analysis of the randomized clinical trial, concentrating on the more complex clinical trial of a disease with many manifestations, and to which many of the problems alluded to in preceding chapters apply. These include postrandomization stratification to account for prognostic variables (possibly with an imbalance), life table analyses in the presence of dropouts, and interim sequential analyses for patient safety data monitoring.

Although the following discussion does not apply to all clinical trials, it displays many of the issues which are potentially present in every clinical trial. A simple randomized clinical trial of two groups using an objective, continuous outcome measure, such as serum cholesterol levels before and after treatment, in which all patients successfully complete the treatment program, and in which there are no other complications of design or execution, poses few statistical problems and could be analyzed straightforwardly. Unfortunately, this is not applicable to many clinical trials.

11.2 OUTCOME EVENTS

By far the most controversial aspect of the analysis of any complex clinical trial rests in the choice of which variables will be analyzed. This is a difficult task and one which requires careful thought and consideration (see Chapters 6 and 10). Although the dependent variables in the statistical analyses are implied directly by the statement of objectives, there is great leeway for interpretation, and the results of a trial may be analyzed many ways, each in some sense being consistent with the objectives. At the most basic level in the evaluation of the results of a clinical trial, one wishes to analyze <u>events</u> of relevance to the objectives, but which events and when?

Categories of Events

In almost every clinical trial it is possible to classify three categories of events: those indicative of efficacy, those indicative of toxicity, and those suggestive of toxicity.

1. <u>Events which indicate efficacy</u> are often the easiest to determine and are best defined on the basis of a direct measure of therapeutic effect, such as ulcer healing demonstrated on endoscopic examination. Indirect measures of efficacy may also be defined, e.g., reduction in gastric secretion, but should not be employed in lieu of an appropriate direct measure (see Chapters 6 and 10).

2. <u>Events which indicate toxicity</u> are those which are related to the toxic effects of the agent employed. Often, any adverse advent is considered to indicate toxicity of the agent, whereas in other cases, based on prior animal research or human experimentation, specific events known to be related to the agent can be defined. Also, any unanticipated event which occurs during follow-up and which disappears during a period of dechallenge and then reappears during a period of rechallenge may be ascribed to the

therapy (even though the patient was known to be receiving placebo). Other adverse effects related to the agent under study, however, may be less obvious, depending on the nature of the disease and the mechanism of action, if known.

3. <u>Events which suggest toxicity</u> are all other adverse events not directly ascribed to the disease under study or the therapy employed. Nevertheless, any seemingly unrelated illness or event should be statistically evaluated as indirectly indicative of potential drug effect. For example, some drugs may induce drowsiness, which could lead to an increased rate of accidents among the treated patients, sometimes leading to accidental death.

Events related to the target disease may be considered in the evaluation either of efficacy or toxicity based on the anticipated therapeutic effects of the agent and knowledge of the natural history of the disease. For almost every disease process, "healing" would obviously be used to assess efficacy. For a multifaceted disease, however, other disease-related events might be classified as reflecting toxicity. For example, in the study of a drug to alleviate angina pectoris in patients with atherosclerotic disease, an increase in cardiovascular mortality would be considered a toxic drug effect.

Dropouts

In defining the various events that will be considered in each of the above categories, an important additional consideration is the act of dropping out of the trial. Patients may drop out of a trial either because they simply become disillusioned, or because they consider themselves cured, or because they have experienced an adverse event. In some trials, dropouts have been removed from all statistical analysis (improperly, see Chapters 4, 6 and 7). More appropriately, they may be treated as censored observations in a life table analysis of one of the other categories of events (such as efficacy). In some cases, however, even this latter approach may not be appropriate, and the act of dropping out might be included among one of the above categories of events.

Timing of the Event

Once the basic events to be analyzed have been defined and categorized, various aspects of the timing of the events must be considered. At issue here is whether the trial is seeking to explore short- versus long-term effects of the therapy. For example, should an event which occurred after termination of therapy, such as myocardial infarction, be counted in the analysis?

In some cases it has also been argued that patients must have been exposed to therapy for some minimum period before events are eligible to be counted in the analysis (1). This is a dangerous practice, however, since patients who exit early from the study for any reason may bias a comparison restricted to events occurring after this minimal exposure period (2). On the other hand, such early events will be equally as likely in all groups if treatment has no effect and inclusion of all patients will be less likely to yield a misleading conclusion.

Some Examples

Perhaps some examples will help to clarify the issues involved. The Coronary Drug Project (3) studied five drugs in comparison to placebo to determine the benefits of each agent in terms of prolonged survival among men with a previous myocardial infarction. This was an 8-year study in which the primary outcome of interest was death. Thus, the indication of efficacy was the survival time of each patient. But which types of deaths should be considered contraindications of efficacy, cardiovascular deaths alone or all deaths? Further, should the analysis be restricted only to death itself, or should it also include other nonfatal cardiovascular events?

In this clinical trial total mortality and cause specific mortality were employed in the analyses, as were all nonfatal cardiovascular-related events (4). Further, for some of the drugs, events indicative of toxicity were also defined (such as gynecomastia due to estrogen) which were also analyzed independently, in fact leading to the termination of three of the agents while the trial was under progress (5-7). All events were analyzed using life table methods, and dropouts were treated as censored observations. A common closing date was employed, and patients were followed for periods up to 8 years.

For such trials in which death is the outcome of interest, the categories of events may be defined straightforwardly. In other trials, this may not be so. The National Cooperative Gallstone Study (8) evaluated the efficacy and safety of chenodeoxycholic acid (a bile acid) in the dissolution of cholesterol gallstones. Obviously, the disappearance of gallstones was the primary event indicative of efficacy.

Two classes of events indicative of toxicity were defined (9). As the gallstones dissolved and became smaller, it was postulated that they might be more likely to leave the gallbladder, obstruct the biliary tract, and cause severe symptoms. The first class of events, therefore, were those related to the disease itself, the outcome event of interest defined to be clinically indicated cholecystectomy (surgical gallbladder removal). Also, prior animal studies had indicated the potential for hepatotoxic reactions to this agent, and thus a second class of events were defined as indications of toxicity due to the drug. These were the need for termination of therapy due to potential liver abnormality as demonstrated by an abnormal liver biopsy or by the recurrence of an elevation of a liver function test following a period of dechallenge and rechallenge. Other severe illnesses unrelated to the drug or the disease were classified as events suggestive of toxicity. Dropouts were treated as censored observations.

In this study, each patient was followed for 2 years, and the principal events were defined as those which occurred at the time of termination of therapy. Thus, the Gallstone Study searched for short-term effects directly due to the agent. The Coronary Drug Project, however, considered all events which occurred up to the closing date regardless of whether the patient had been actively participating in the trial and under therapy. Thus, the emphasis was on long-term effects.

Another difference lies in the direction of the anticipated effects. In the Coronary Drug Project, death was the event indicative of either efficacy or toxicity, depending on whether survival in the treated groups improved or deteriorated as compared to placebo. Since a difference in either direction was clinically relevant, two-sided tests were employed. In the NCGS, one-sided tests were employed for efficacy since differences in one direction only were considered clinically relevant.

These examples point out that in many clinical trials there are a multiplicity of outcome events of interest which can be evaluated in many ways relative to the objectives of the trial and their temporal relationship to the time of randomization into the study, or exit from the study.

11.3 PROGNOSTIC VARIABLES

Previous chapters have stressed the importance of postrandomization stratification in analyses of the results of a clinical trial, the main consideration being the influence of prognostic or baseline variables on the various outcome events of interest. The issue is whether an imbalance in the composition of the treatment groups for a prognostic variable could in turn account for any differences observed between the treatment groups. For example, suppose there is an imbalance in the percentage of females in each of the two treatment groups, say 35% of those in the first group versus 60% of those in the second. If females were better responders than males, the group with the higher proportion of females (the second group) might display a higher percentage of success than the first group just because it contained a higher proportion of females. Thus, the treatment comparison should be adjusted for the imbalance in this prognostic variable.

A related issue in prognostic stratification is to describe the probability of efficacy or toxicity within each stratum to aid the practicing physician in determining the probabilities of success or failure in the treatment of an individual future patient. Our primary interest here shall be the adjustment of treatment effects for prognostic variables, although the latter issue will also be discussed.

A first step in the statistical analysis should be to examine the composition of the treatment groups for those prognostic variables known or suspected to be related to one or more of the various outcomes of interest, those related to either efficacy or toxicity. The composition of the treatment groups for the various prognostic variables should be examined closely, and the safest approach is to consider even a slight imbalance to be potentially important in the evaluation of the effects of treatment. Often, formal statistical tests of the differences between the groups are conducted, but these may serve as a poor guideline for the selection of prognostic variables. Whether a difference of 35% females in one group versus 60% in the other will be statistically significant depends on the sample size employed in the clinical trial. If an imbalance of this extent were to occur, however, it would be mandatory that confounding of patient sex with the effects of treatment effect be explored, regardless of whether the imbalance itself was declared statistically significant.

11.4 MANTEL-HAENSZEL PROCEDURE

One of the most widely employed methods of statistical analysis in clinical trials is the Mantel-Haenszel procedure (10-12), which provides an adjusted evaluation of treatment effect (drug-placebo difference) over the various strata of a prognostic variable or multiple prognostic variables. For example, consider again the hypothetical data presented in Table 5.2 of two separate clinical trials conducted in countries A and B which studied the efficacy of an antisecretory agent in the treatment of gastric ulcer. In each study, the patients were stratified postrandomization according to ulcer type I, II, or III. The data are presented again in a slightly different format as Table 11.1

These data were presented in Chapter 5 to illustrate the importance of patient selection criteria and their potential effects on the eventual outcome of the clinical trial. It was pointed out that the type I ulcers tended to be nonresponders, and thus the clinical trial conducted in country B with a lower prevalence of type I ulcers produced a significant treatment-control difference, whereas that conducted in country A with a high prevalence of type I ulcers failed to produce a significant effect. In both these hypothetical studies, however, important information was ignored by failing to incorporate the prognostic stratification by ulcer type in the overall analysis of treatment effect.

Within each ulcer type stratum a 2 x 2 contingency table can be constructed

(1)

in stratum i	Drug	Placebo	
Healed	A_i	B_i	M_{1i}
Not healed	C_i	D_i	M_{2i}
	N_{1i}	N_{2i}	T_i

from which a continuity-corrected chi-square test, χ_i^2, with one degree of freedom can be calculated,

(2)
$$\chi_i^2 = \frac{T_i(|A_i D_i - B_i C_i| - \tfrac{1}{2}T_i)^2}{N_{1i} N_{2i} M_{1i} M_{2i}}$$

in order to test the hypothesis that drug and placebo have equal effect

TABLE 11.1 Mantel-Haenszel Analysis of Hypothetical Data from Two Clinical Trials of Ulcer Healing Presented in Table 5.2

	Sample sizes			No. healed on drug			Chi square (1 df)	Odds ratio (95% limits)
	Total (T_i)	Drug (N_{1i})	Placebo (N_{2i})	Obs. (A_i)	Exp. (E_i)	Var. (V_i)		
Country A								
Type I	89	42	47	16	16.99	5.40	0.04	0.83 (0.15-4.63)
Type II	21	12	9	9	7.43	1.27	0.95	3.75 (0.26-53.76)
Type III	90	46	44	28	22.49	5.68	4.47	2.72 (1.08-6.89)
Sum (Σ)	200	100	100	53	46.91	12.36	$\chi_a^2=2.53$	1.63 (0.89-2.99)
Country B								
Type I	31	17	14	6	6.58	1.88	0.004	0.73 (<0.01 - >99.9)
Type II	138	68	70	47	36.46	8.64	11.74	3.56 (1.72-7.37)
Type III	31	15	16	7	6.77	1.98	0.001	1.13 (0.35-3.61)
Sum (Σ)	200	100	100	60	49.82	12.50	$\chi_a^2=7.50$	2.27 (1.26-4.07)
Sum (Σ) over both countries	400	200	200	113	96.73	24.86	$\chi_a^2=10.00$	1.92 (1.28-2.88)

on the healing rate. The extent of treatment effect within each stratum is measured by the odds ratio

(3) $$R_i = \frac{A_i D_i}{B_i C_i}$$

which is simply the odds of healing when treated with drug A_i/C_i relative to that when treated with placebo B_i/D_i. The X_i^2 test is equivalent to the test that the population odds ratio within that stratum is unity, i.e,. that there are equal odds of healing when treated with drug or placebo. Denoting the true population odds ratio as Ω, Miettinen (13) has proposed that an approximate $(1-\alpha)\%$ confidence interval on $\omega = \ln \Omega$ be obtained from

(4) $$(1 \pm \frac{Z_{\alpha/2}}{X}) \ln R$$

where $Z_{\alpha/2}$ is the two-sided critical value for the standard normal distribution (see Chapter 9) and X is the square root of the value of the chi-square statistic obtained from Eq. (2). Denoting an obtained interval as $u \leq \omega \leq v$, the corresponding $(1-\alpha)\%$ confidence interval on the odds ratio Ω is given by $e^u \leq \Omega \leq e^v$.

Fleiss (14) shows that the above confidence interval is the most accurate among those readily calculable directly, but as shown by others, tends to be too narrow as compared to the exact interval based on Fisher's exact test for 2 x 2 tables. For more accurate calculations, Fleiss (14) recommends an iterative calculation based on the earlier work of Cornfield (15).

As an illustration, the above methods may be applied to the 2 x 2 tables separately within each of the three ulcer strata for the clinical trials in countries A and B, with results presented in Table 11.1. Among the three ulcer strata in country A, drug treatment yields a significantly greater proportion healed than does placebo only for type III ulcers. What is required, however, is a pooled test of drug effectiveness over all three ulcer strata in country A, yet adjusting for the imbalances in the numbers of patients in the treatment groups within each stratum.

Because the chi-square test within each stratum is based on one degree of freedom, attention can be focused on only one cell of each table without any true loss of information. Within each stratum consider the observed numbers A_i of patients treated with drug who healed, shown in Table 11.1. Within each stratum, the expected number of drug-treated patients who would have been expected to heal if the drug and placebo had equal effect is $E_i = N_{1i}M_{1i}/T_i$. The variance of the observed frequency is

$$(5) \quad V_i = \frac{N_{1i}N_{2i}M_{1i}M_{2i}}{T_i^2(T_i - 1)}$$

These quantities A_i, E_i, and V_i are then summed across the s strata (s = 3 in this case) and the sums employed in the following equation to yield the Mantel-Haenszel chi-square statistic on one degree of freedom:

$$(6) \quad \chi_a^2 = \frac{(|\Sigma_i A_i - \Sigma_i E_i| - \frac{1}{2})^2}{\Sigma_i V_i}$$

The contingency χ^2 statistic in Eq. (2) requires that the sample size T be large enough that no expected value for any of the four observed frequencies be less than 5. Mantel and Fleiss (16), however, have suggested that the Mantel-Haenszel statistic in Eq. (6) is valid provided that both

$$(7) \quad \begin{array}{l} \Sigma_i E_i - \Sigma_i A_{i(L)} \geq 5 \\ \Sigma_i E_i - \Sigma_i A_{i(H)} \geq 5 \end{array}$$

where within each stratum the $A_{i(L)}$ and $A_{i(H)}$ are the lowest and highest possible values for A_i given the marginal totals, i.e.,

$$A_{i(L)} = \max(0, M_{1i} - N_{2i})$$
$$A_{i(H)} = \min(N_{1i}, M_{1i})$$

Thus, the Mantel-Haenszel statistic may be valid even though the minimum expected value within a stratum is less than 5.

The Mantel-Haenszel statistic has been called a test of <u>partial association</u> between treatment (drug versus placebo) and outcome (healed versus not healed) since it provides a test of treatment differences pooled over strata and adjusting for the influence of the stratification variable (17, 18). The summary measure of treatment effect pooled over strata is then expressed by the summary adjusted odds ratio

$$(8) \quad R_a = \frac{\Sigma_i (A_i D_i / T_i)}{\Sigma_i (B_i C_i / T_i)}$$

Approximate $(1-\alpha)\%$ confidence limits can then be obtained from Eq. (4) using the adjusted odds ratio R_a and chi-square statistic χ_a^2 from the Mantel-Haenszel procedure.

As shown in Table 11.1, accounting for the ulcer strata yields a total of 53 patients healed when treated with drug ($\Sigma_i A_i$), with a pooled expected number of patients healed $\Sigma_i E_i = 46.97$, and a pooled variance $\Sigma_i V_i = 12.36$. This yields an adjusted chi-square value $\chi_a^2 = 2.53$ with a p-value of 0.11. Thus, stratification by ulcer type in the analysis provides less evidence for a treatment effect than was provided by the original analysis in Table 5.2, ignoring ulcer strata.

Closer examination of the data indicates the reason for this reduction in the value of the chi-square test of treatment effect. Since type I ulcers are nonresponders, and since the drug-treated group contained 42% type I ulcers versus 47% among the placebo group, then the drug group would tend to display a higher percentage healed than the placebo group due to this slight imbalance. In the Mantel-Haenszel procedure, however, drug is compared to placebo within each ulcer stratum and then the results are pooled. In this case imbalances between the treatment groups within each stratum no longer bias the comparison.

Applying the Mantel-Haenszel procedure to the clinical trial conducted in country B, the adjusted chi-square value is $\chi_a^2 = 7.50$, which is again highly significant. In this trial, however, there was a slightly higher proportion of nonresponders in the drug-treated group which would tend to artifically lower the observed healing response within the drug group as a whole. Again, this is accounted for by prognostic stratification, yielding an adjusted chi-square statistic which is slightly increased above that previously observed, ignoring ulcer strata.

The effects of adjustment can also be illustrated by comparing the estimated odds ratios and their 95% confidence intervals, ignoring prognostic stratification versus accounting for prognostic stratification. In country A, R = 1.69 (0.92 - 3.10), ignoring strata, while $R_a = 1.63$ (0.89 - 2.99), taking account of stratification. Conversely, in country B, R = 2.25 (1.25 - 4.07), while $R_a = 2.27$ (1.26 - 4.07). This example illustrates that in some instances, prognostic stratification will increase the values for the estimated odds ratio and the observed chi-square statistic, whereas in other cases it will decrease. Although this example demonstrates only slight differences between the unadjusted and adjusted analyses, in cases in which there is a greater degree of imbalance for a prognostic variable, the differences may be substantial.

This procedure can also be extended indefinitely to account for a variety of prognostic strata simultaneously. For example, an overall evaluation of the drug in comparison to placebo can be obtained using the evidence provided by both studies, in this case with stratification both by country of origin and ulcer type, six strata in all. Combining both studies, there are 113 patients observed to heal when treated with the drug with a pooled expectation totaling 96.73 yielding an estimated odds ratio $R_a = 1.92$ (1.28 - 2.88) and an adjusted $\chi_a^2 = 10.0$ on one degree of freedom, providing overwhelming evidence of the efficacy of the drug.

This latter analysis points to the power of the Mantel-Haenszel procedure. Not only does the procedure compare treatments within strata, it builds upon the evidence across strata. Assuming that treatment has no effect, drug would be expected to be better than control by chance alone in some strata, and control to be better in others. If, however, drug treatment is consistently better than control across strata, i.e., is homogeneous, the Mantel-Haenszel statistic will likely be greater than the unstratified χ^2, and thus is more likely to be declared statistically significant.*

In fact, when the treatment effect (the odds ratio) is homogeneous within strata, the adjusted χ_a^2 may become as large as, but algebraically cannot exceed, the sum of the individual χ_i^2 within strata. Thus, for example, $\chi_a^2 = 10.0$ with stratification by country and ulcer type, whereas the sum of the χ_i^2 for the 6 individual strata is 17.21. As would be expected, however, when the treatment effect within the say s strata is heterogeneous, the adjusted χ_a^2 will be much smaller than the $\Sigma_i \chi_i^2$ over strata. This fact has lead to the suggestion that the difference $\chi_d^2 = \Sigma_i \chi_i^2 - \chi_a^2$ be used as a χ^2 test for homogeneity on s - 1 df (19). For the data in Table 11.1, this latter test for homogeneity yields $\chi_d^2 = 7.2$ on 5 df, which is not significant (p < 0.20). This test, however, may be misleading and should generally be avoided (20,21). Rather, it is preferable that a direct test of interaction in the multiway table be conducted (20,22) to assess heterogeneity; which for the data in Table 5.2 yields $\chi^2 = 10.10$, p = 0.08.

In summary, the Mantel-Haenszel procedure provides a powerful method for adjusting the treatment comparison for any imbalances

---

*When the treatment effect is relatively homogeneous among strata, the Mantel-Haenszel statistic Eq. (6) will have greater power than the unstratified statistic Eq. (2), which is equivalent to the test of two proportions, the power function for which is presented in Chapter 9. The power of the Mantel-Haenszel statistic has been described by Birch (17) and is a function of the odds ratio within each stratum and the marginal sample sizes.

between the treatment groups within strata based on prognostic variables. Such poststratification in the data analysis reduces the need for stratified randomization (prerandomization stratification). Further, since similar clinical trials conducted in the same patient population by different investigators can be considered as additional strata, as was done with the clinical trials from countries A and B above, the Mantel-Haenszel procedure also provides the most appropriate procedure for combining results from many similar clinical trials.

Although the above presentation is based on the evaluation of the simple 2 x 2 table across various strata, the Mantel-Haenszel procedure has been generalized to the evaluation of r x c tables across strata (18). The calculation of this adjusted chi-square statistic, χ_a^2, for the test of partial association in r x c tables over strata involves matrix operations not amenable to hand calculation. In their original paper, however, Mantel and Haenszel (10) present a direct solution for 2 x 3 tables (e.g., two outcomes and three treatment groups) over s strata.

11.5 THE ACTUARIAL LIFE TABLE METHOD

Among the most useful methods of analysis for clinical trials is the life table method which considers not only whether the outcome event occurred, but <u>when</u> during treatment it occurred. The life table method was originally developed for use by actuaries to describe the cumulative proportion of survivors after t years of follow-up in a cohort, i.e., a defined group of individuals, only a few of whom may actually have been observed for the full t years. In a clinical trial, survivorship simply refers to failure to reach a <u>terminal event</u>, such as death, healing, or other clinical outcome. The method is based on the statistical principles of conditional probability whereby all individuals entering a time interval contribute information about the survivorship function during that interval, and thus over the period of observation up to that point in time. In this manner, each individual contributes to the analysis over the period of time he was actually observed, even though the individual may be censored, i.e., lost to follow-up, before being observed to reach the terminal event. This feature is most important to clinical trials in which not all patients have been followed for the full term. The method is lucidly described by Cutler and Ederer (23).

To illustrate the method, the clinical trials in countries A and B above are again employed, with consideration for the period of observation of each patient. First, assume that patients were examined endoscopically at 4, 8, and 12 weeks after initiation of therapy to evaluate whether each patient still had an ulcer at each point in time, with those patients found not to have an ulcer at each examination considered healed (the terminal event) and withdrawn from further therapy. Second, assume that some of the patients either discontinued follow-up, dropped out, or were withdrawn from the study for other serious illnesses, i.e., observation was censored. Further, assume that all patients censored were examined endoscopically and that none were found to have healed (otherwise the patient would be considered healed, not censored). Third, assume that censored observations would have displayed the same healing (terminal event) rate as all other patients had they remained under follow-up.

Thus, not all patients were observed for the full 12 weeks of study. The prior analyses, however, considered only the crude proportions healed among all those randomized within each group. These studies, however, could also be analyzed using the life table method, which would incorporate the added information concerning the proportions healed at each of the three examinations.

Calculating the Actuarial Life Table

The life table is based on the measure of the trial time t_i for the ith patient. In a clinical trial, the trial time t_i for the ith patient is simply the time elapsed from the day of randomization of that patient to the last day of observation of that patient, i.e., to the time of the terminal event or censoring, or if neither, to the end of the study period of follow-up.

Statistical Analysis   171

For a fixed maximum length follow-up schedule (see Chapter 7), the last day of observation for each patient will not exceed the maximum length of the study (12 weeks in this case). Under a common closing date follow-up schedule, some patients may achieve trial times up to the maximum attainable (the number of days elapsed from the randomization of the first patient to the common closing date). For both types of follow-up schedules the analysis is conducted in the same manner. The only difference is that with a common closing date, a patient's trial time may be censored for the added reason that the patient was only followed for time t_i when the common closing date was reached. Such patients are often termed <u>administrative withdrawals</u>.

From these trial times for all patients, the proportions healed within desired time intervals then can be calculated. Consider the data from the drug-treated group in country A as shown in Table 11.2, ignoring ulcer type. Since endoscopic examinations are conducted at 4-week intervals, three time intervals are employed: 0 to 4, 5 to 8, and 9 to 12 weeks respectively. For each time interval, a separate stratum is constructed within which are presented:

L_i = the number entering the ith interval
d_i = the number observed to have reached the terminal event (healing) during that interval
W_i = the number censored, i.e., lost to follow-up or withdrawn from study during the interval.

The number exposed to "healing" during each interval is then determined, of which the proportion healed during the interval is obtained. In calculating this proportion healed, censored observations W_i are assumed to have been observed for half the interval on the average, and for each interval, therefore, the number exposed to healing is expressed as $N_i = L_i - \frac{1}{2}W_i$. From this, the conditional probability of healing during the interval is calculated as $q_i = d_i/N_i$, or simply

TABLE 11.2 Life Table of the Cumulative Proportion Not Healed in the Drug Treated Group from the Clinical Trial in Country A Ignoring Ulcer Strata

Time interval (i)	No. entering interval (L_{1i})	No. healed (d_{1i})	No. censored (W_{1i})	No. exposed (N_{1i})	Proportion healed (q_{1i})	Cumulative proportion not healed (P_{1i})	S.E. (P_{1i})
0-4 weeks	100	16	6	97	0.165	0.835	0.038
>4-8 weeks	78	25	3	76.5	0.327	0.562	0.051
>8-12 weeks	50	12	1	49.5	0.242	0.426	0.052
Totals		53	10				

$$q_i = \frac{\text{number entering and who heal during the ith interval}}{\text{number exposed to healing during the ith interval}}$$

What is desired, however, is an estimate of the cumulative proportion healed after 12 weeks which would have been observed had all patients been followed for the full 12-week period of observation except for those previously healed. Within the context of a life table, this is equivalent to estimating the cumulative survivorship function, in this case the cumulative proportion not healed. Given the proportions healed within each interval, the cumulative survivorship (not healed) function after the ith interval can be estimated as

(9) $\qquad P_i = (1 - q_i)P_{i-1}$

which is simply the probability $(1 - q_i)$ of not healing in the ith interval given that one did not heal earlier times the probability (P_{i-1}) of not healing earlier. For example, after three intervals

(10) $\qquad \begin{aligned} P_3 &= (1 - q_3)P_2 \\ &= (1 - q_3)(1 - q_2)P_1 \\ &= (1 - q_3)(1 - q_2)(1 - q_1) \end{aligned}$

Thus, the cumulative proportion not healed after 12 weeks of therapy can be expressed as the product of the conditional probabilities of not healing, the $1 - q_i$, for each interval. The life table estimate of the cumulative proportion not healed after 12 weeks, 0.426, is thus obtained as the product $(1 - 0.165)(1 - 0.327)(1 - 0.242)$. The cumulative proportion healed is then estimated to be $(1 - 0.426) = 0.574$. This is slightly higher than the crude proportion 0.53 which had been observed previously, which in effect ignored the censored observations.

The standard error of the estimated cumulative proportion of survivors after each interval then can be obtained by the Greenwood formula (see Ref. 23) as

(11) $\qquad SE(P_i) = P_i \left[\sum_{j=1}^{i} \frac{q_j}{N_j - d_j} \right]^{1/2}$

Advantages of the Life Table Method

There are two principal advantages of the life table method. The first is that censored observations contribute to the analysis over those intervals of time they were followed. The six censored observations during the first interval in Table 11.2 were assumed to have been followed for half the interval, and the other four censored observations that occurred in later intervals contributed fully to the analysis through the first time interval, and partly during later intervals.

In many clinical trials, however, it is not possible to conduct an examination for the terminal event at the time of censoring for all censored observations. This is especially important in those trials in which reaching an outcome event is contingent upon the conduct of a procedure (e.g., endoscopy) which censored observations may not undergo at the time of censoring. Denote as W_i' those censored observations during interval i where it is impossible to know whether they had reached the terminal event at the time of censoring. In this case, the number exposed in each interval is calculated as $N_i = L_i - \frac{1}{2} W_i - W_i'$. All censored observations with unknown status W_i' are removed from consideration since their status is assumed last known at the time last observed.

The second advantage of the life table method is that it incorporates in the analysis the time to the outcome event for each patient. Table 11.3 presents the cumulative proportion not healed (P_i) for both the drug and placebo groups. In both groups, approximately 10% of the patients were censored (W_i) and the rate of censoring over the time intervals is comparable for the two groups. Under the latter condition it is then appropriate to compare the cumulative proportions not healed (or healed) among the two groups. During the first 4 weeks 17% healed in the drug-treated group (versus 6% for placebo), whereas the majority of the placebo-healed ulcers were observed during the interval 8 to 12 weeks. Thus, even though the overall crude proportions healed within each group (ignoring time) were not significant in the

TABLE 11.3 Life Table Estimates of the Cumulative Proportion Healed in the Drug and Placebo Groups from the Clinical Trial in Country A

Time interval (1)	Drug (group 1)					Placebo (group 2)				
	N_{1i}[a]	d_{1i}	W_{1i}	q_{1i}	P_{1i}	N_{2i}	d_{2i}	W_{2i}	q_{2i}	P_{2i}
0-4 weeks	97	16	6	0.165	0.835	97.5	6	5	0.062	0.938
>4-8 weeks	76.5	25	3	0.327	0.526	87.5	12	3	0.137	0.809
>8-12 weeks	49.5	12	1	0.242	0.426	73	22	2	0.301	0.566
Totals		53	10				40	10		

[a]The number entering each interval is $L_{1i} = N_{1i} + \frac{1}{2}W_{1i}$.

previous analysis, the groups appear to be different in the observed timing of healing.

Test of Group Differences

The differences in the healing rate in the two groups across time can be tested using the same Mantel-Haenszel procedure described above, in which the three time intervals are treated as separate strata. For each time interval a 2 x 2 table is constructed similar to Eq. (1) with the entries obtained from the drug and placebo life tables:

(12)

In interval i	Drug	Placebo	
Healed	$A_i = d_{1i}$	$B_i = d_{2i}$	M_{1i}
Not healed	$C_i = N_{1i} - d_{1i}$	$D_i = N_{2i} - d_2$	M_{2i}
	N_{1i}	N_{2i}	

Applying the Mantel-Haenszel procedure to Table 11.3 yields the aggregate chi-square statistic $\chi_a^2 = 16.79$ on 1 df, $p < 0.001$.

In this example, the simple proportions of ulcers healed in the two groups were not significantly different, but the Mantel-Haenszel statistic comparing the life tables declared a highly significant difference because ulcers healed faster in the drug-treated group. In general, the Mantel-Haenszel procedure, when applied to the comparison of life tables, is sensitive to a difference between the groups in the time to healing and not only to the cumulative proportions of events at the end of the study.

The Mantel-Haenszel procedure could also be employed to compare the two life tables adjusting for the ulcer strata by establishing three time interval strata within each of the three ulcer strata, nine strata in all. Within each stratum separate life tables are constructed for each treatment group and the groups compared by means of the adjusted Mantel-Haenszel statistic calculated over the nine strata.

Censored Observations

Prior to constructing a life table and conducting a treatment group comparison, it is important to consider the potential effects of censoring. These life table methods and the Mantel-Haenszel test assume, respectively, that

1. Censored observations would have displayed the same event rate as noncensored observations had they not been censored, i.e., that they are <u>unbiased</u>.
2. Censoring is not related to the effects of treatment.

Neither assumption is testable directly but each may be examined by indirect means. For each characteristic of the patient population, i.e., prognostic variable, the proportion (and timing) of censored observations could be compared. For example, did censoring occur at a higher rate or sooner among males than it did among females? If so, and if females responded differently to the drug therapy, then the first assumption would not be tenable and the cumulative life table estimate would be biased. Likewise, the rate of censoring in each group could be compared, and if different, might suggest a violation of the second assumption.

To demonstrate the effects of a violation of these assumptions, assume that the rate of censoring in the drug-treated group had been 30 patients of 100, rather than 10, with W_{li} three times those shown in Table 11.2. Further, assume that those who dropped out were different from those who continued under follow-up, and that none would have been healed had they continued (i.e., they are biased). Since the number healed would be the same as that shown in Table 11.2, the cumulative proportion not healed after 12 weeks would then have become only 30% (70% healed) rather than the 43% observed above. Thus, prior to conducting a statistical test comparing the life tables for the various treatment groups it first must be demonstrated that the overall proportion and timing of censored observations is comparable between the groups.

This can be accomplished by constructing a life table in which censoring is employed as the terminal event and the healed observations are treated as censored at the time of healing. In each interval the number exposed is calculated as $N_i = L_i - \frac{1}{2}d_i$, and the proportion censored calculated as $q_i = W_i/N_i$. The Mantel-Haenszel procedure then could be used to test whether the proportion and timing of dropouts in the two groups are equivalent.

If it is found that either of the above assumptions are not tenable, i.e., censored observations may be biased or the rate of censoring is not comparable among the groups, then the safest method of analysis is simply to employ crude proportions as had been done in Tables 5.2 and 11.2.

11.6 THE PRODUCT LIMIT METHOD AND THE LOG RANK TEST

In the previous example, the trial times, i.e., the times to healing, were only measured approximately, since patients were examined periodically to assess healing. The life table in such a situation is often termed a life table in <u>grouped time</u> due to grouping of the time measures. In a study of true survival (or mortality), however, each patient is at risk of the terminal event at each point in time. In this case, it is possible to measure the time to the terminal event exactly for each patient, and to construct a life table using the successive exact times at which each patient encounters the event. Because there is no grouping of the time measures, such a life table is often referred to as a life table in <u>continuous time</u>, a product limit, or a Kaplan-Meier (24) life table.

In a continuous time life table, each patient's trial time to the terminal event or censoring is usually measured in days since randomization. As before, patients who were withdrawn from follow-up (including administrative withdrawals) or dropped out are assumed known to be alive at the time of censoring and are assumed to be unbiased. The life table is then presented in like manner to Table 11.3 but with the distinct trial times of the successive terminal events forming separate strata in ascending sequence. Thus, the patients with the shortest trial times appear first in the table, while those with the longest trial times appear last. Strata are not constructed for those trial times at which only withdrawal or dropping out occurred.

In such a table, on any given day the number N_i at risk of the event would be the same as the number L_i of patients still under follow-up at the beginning of that day, and the number d_i of terminal events during the day would be as observed. Censored observations do not come into play, since $N_i = L_i$, and no adjustment is made to the denominator in calculating the proportion of events within each interval. For example, suppose that one patient encountered the event on day 220 and the next patient to encounter the event did so on day 232. Further assume that a patient dropped out on day 225. This dropout would be included in the number at risk in the life table entry at day 220, but would not be included in the next life table entry at day 232. There would be no life table entry for day 225.

The product limit life table estimate of the cumulative proportion surviving after an interval (trial time) is obtained as the product of the proprotion of survivors in that interval times the cumulative estimate for the prior interval, exactly as for the actuarial life table. In the limit, i.e., if the sample size were to become infinite and events were then to be incurred at each successive day, these estimates would describe the exact survival distribution whatever its form.

The equality of the survival distributions of the treated and control groups is then tested using the Mantel-Haenszel procedure as described above. If in fact only one patient was observed to have encountered the terminal event on a given day, then within the 2 x 2 table for that stratum (day) only one of the two groups would show an event at that time; the other none, i.e., either A_i or B_i, would equal 1 in the 2 x 2 table shown as Eq. (12). In this case the expected number E_i of events in the treated group would be a fraction (0.50 if the numbers at risk in each group on that day are equal). These expectations are often termed the extents of exposure. Even though the E_i will be a fraction for most strata, the test statistic usually is valid since in Eq. (7) the $A_{i(L)} = 0$ and $A_{i(H)} = M_{1i}$ for all strata (except possibly the last).

The Mantel-Haenszel test statistic applied to a product limit life table is termed the <u>log rank test</u> (25) because the separate strata in the life table are defined according to the order in which the terminal events occur and not the specific times at which they occur. In this context the Mantel-Haenszel statistic becomes a rank order statistic. Other statistical tests have also been developed for the comparison of life table survival curves; however, the Mantel-Haenszel procedure is optimally efficient under general conditions.

The Mantel-Haenszel procedure (log rank test) could also be employed to adjust for a prognostic variable exactly as described above for the actuarial life table. Separate product limit life tables are constructed within each level of the prognostic variable, and the Mantel-Haenszel statistic calculated by summing entries over time and levels of the prognostic variable. Thus, apart from the feature of continuous time, the analysis is identical to the actuarial life table method. An excellent example of the continuous time life table, and a discussion of some of the finer statistical considerations in the log rank test, are presented by Peto et al. (26).

For the comparison of survival times among more than two groups, the log rank test, as does the test of partial association, involves matrix operations which are not amenable to hand calculation. Peto and Pike (27), however, have presented an accurate approximation which may be applied when trial times of terminal events are nearly distinct, i.e., when there are few ties.

Within each stratum i, that is, at each time of a terminal event, the observed number of events for each of g treatment groups is denoted as $O_{j(i)}$ with $M_i = \sum_{j=1}^{g} O_{j(i)}$ being the total number of events at the ith time, M_i being only 1 (i.e., only one event) for most intervals. With $N_{j(i)}$ denoting the number of patients in the jth group entering the ith interval, and $T_i = \sum_{j=1}^{g} N_{j(i)}$, then the extent of exposure for group j at that time is obtained as $E_{j(i)} = N_{j(i)} M_i / T_i$. The observed events and extents of exposure in each group are then summed and these sums employed to calculate an approximate log rank statistic

(13)
$$\chi^2_{a'} = \sum_{j=1}^{g} \frac{\left[\sum_i O_{j(i)} - \sum_i E_{j(i)}\right]^2}{\sum_i E_{j(i)}}$$

which is approximately distributed as chi-square on $g - 1$ degrees of freedom.

11.7 SUBGROUP ANALYSES

Types of Subgroup Analyses

The phrase subgroup analyses has been employed in various contexts to refer to at least three distinct classes of analyses.

1. The comparison of treatment groups may be adjusted for imbalances in the composition of the groups on one or more prognostic variables, as described above using the Mantel-Haenszel procedure.
2. The effects of the treatment can be compared across the different levels of a prognostic variable, for example, to determine whether there is a higher healing rate among type I ulcers than type II ulcers within the drug-treated group.
3. The treatments may be compared within a specific subgroup of patients, for example, to determine whether the healing rate in the drug-treated group is higher than that for placebo specifically within type I ulcers.

Note that in the second class the strata are compared within a treatment group, while in the third class the treatment groups are compared within strata.

As an example of the second class of subgroup analyses, within the drug treatment group of the study from country A in Table 11.1, a 2 x 3 contingency table of healed or not healed versus ulcer type could be formed. A contingency chi-square test on two degrees of freedom then could be conducted comparing the proportions healed among type I, type

II, and type III ulcers to determine whether ulcer type has any influence on the healing rate within the drug-treated group. Likewise, a separate chi-square test could be conducted within the placebo-treated group comparing the proportions healed among the three ulcer types. The Mantel-Haenszel procedure then could be employed comparing healing among type I, type II, and type III ulcers, adjusting for the effects of treatment, by summing the observed and expected frequencies and variances over the two treatment groups to obtain an aggregate Mantel-Haenszel statistic. A similar analysis could also be employed using life tables, in which the life tables are compared among subgroups, either within a treatment group of interest or in aggregate over the treatment groups using the Mantel-Haenszel summary chi-square statistic. For this example, the generalized Mantel-Haenszel procedure for comparing more than two conditions would be employed as described in Ref. 18 or 25.

The third and potentially most misleading class of subgroup analyses is the comparison of treatment group differences within subgroups. For example, in describing the Mantel-Haenszel procedure for the ulcer-healing trial conducted in country A, a separate contingency table chi-square statistic comparing drug to placebo within each ulcer stratum was calculated in Table 11.1. These separate chi-square statistics were presented in order to demonstrate the relative homogeneity among the different ulcer strata. Such analyses within strata have also been employed to identify subgroups within which treatment is superior to controls, often examining various combinations of prognostic variables, such as the subgroup of patients with type III ulcers who are also nonsmokers and nondrinkers. However, when examining a variety of prognostic variables, separately or in combination, with a moderate sample size, one is likely by chance alone to be able to identify some specific subgroup of patients within which treatment is significantly different from control. Such analyses, therefore, should be regarded with suspicion, especially if a treatment group difference is not demonstrated for all patients combined, or if specific subgroups were not identified a priori.

Protecting Type I Error

For the first class of subgroup analyses, no specific precautions are needed, since the Mantel-Haenszel summary statistic by its nature will adjust the treatment comparison for heterogeneity among the different strata. In the second and third classes, however, the type I error α increases with the number of comparisons conducted among or within subgroups. In these types of anlayses, the nominal α level employed can be adjusted in order to guarantee that the true type I error level does not exceed some specified amount. Using the improved Bonferroni inequality (28), if k subgroup comparisons are to be conducted, the nominal α level

(14) $$\alpha' = 1 - (1 - \alpha)^{1/k}$$

could be employed in order to achieve a true type I error not exceeding α. For example, if 20 subgroup comparisons are to be conducted in this manner, then each could be tested at nominal signifinance level α' = 0.0026 in order to ensure an overall type I error level of α = 0.05 for the 20 comparisons.

Of course, this assumes that the subgroup comparisons to be conducted were specified beforehand and not on the basis of examination of the data. In the latter case, no statistical procedure can be employed to guard against the inflation of the type I error which is incurred. Also, this implies that only a small number of subgroup comparisons should be planned. As the number of comparisons increases, the nominal α level employed decreases disproportionately, thus making it more difficult to achieve significance.

Confounding and Censoring

In conducting subgroup analyses, one must also be careful to consider the effects of confounding and censoring. It is likely that two prognostic variables which are highly correlated will show similar subgroup effects. For example, suppose that females were found to have a significantly higher rate of ulcer healing when treated with drug than did males. Since females tend to be smaller than males, then if patients were grouped according to body weight (such as those above and below the median), it might be found that those with lower body weight also show a significantly higher rate of healing than those with higher body weight. However, those with lower body weight tend predominately to be female, and thus the two effects are confounded. It is difficult from such analyses, therefore, to infer causation.

Further, even though the proportion of dropouts and withdrawals might be equal within the drug and placebo groups, subgroup comparisons may be grossly affected by differences in the characteristics of the dropouts versus those of nondropouts. For example, assume that dropouts occurred at a much higher rate among females than had occurred among males. (Thus, dropouts also occurred at a higher rate among those with low body weight.) Also, assume that the agent was equally effective in males and females, but that the females who dropped out are the same patients for whom the agent would not have been efficacous. Thus, the female dropouts are biased. If the rates of healing within the drug-treated group among males and females were compared using the life table method, then the higher proportion of female dropouts will result in a lowered number at risk, and thus a higher estimated proportion of females healed among those actually followed. Thus, the higher rate of censoring among females in the life table analysis might likely lead to a significant difference between males and females in the proportions healed, even though the agent is equally effective for both. In such cases, therefore, it is best to employ crude proportions to account for the potential effects of differential censoring within the subgroups.

11.8 THE LOGISTIC REGRESSION MODEL

Just as simple direct methods of analysis, such as the Mantel-Haenszel procedure, can be employed for the examination of subgroup effects, so also may a regression model. For example, Truett et al. (29) applied a logistic regression model to predict the risk of heart failure on the basis of a set of prognostic variables. Similar analyses have been conducted in clinical trials in which a logistic regression model is constructed to predict the risk of the outcome event among the patients in the drug-treated group on the basis of a set of prognostic variables. In this regard, the regression model is an extension of the third class of subgroup analyses described above.

The Regression Model

Under the logistic regression model, the probability p of an event of interest (such as healing) is expressed as a function of k prognostic variables $X_1, \ldots, X_k$ through the logit relationship

$$\ln \frac{p}{1-p} = \beta_0 + \sum_{i=1}^{k} \beta_i X_i \tag{15}$$

The regression coefficients $(\beta_0, \beta_1, \ldots, \beta_k)$ in this model and their standard errors can be estimated assuming multivariate normality or using an iterative maximum likelihood procedure (see Ref. 30, Chapter 6). Computationally, the coefficients are more easily obtained under the assumption of multivariate normality, but this assumption will not apply in the event that discrete prognostic variables are included in the model. Conversely, the iterative maximum likelihood procedure requires no such assumptions on the joint distribution of the predictors. For a discrete prognostic variable with m categories, such as marital status with three categories (never married, married, or previously married), separate binary (i.e., 0 or 1) indicator variables for m - 1 of the categories can be constructed, taking the value 1 when that category applies, and 0 otherwise. For the marital status variable, two indicator variables could be established for never married and married, respectively. Only two variables are needed, since the value 0 for both variables in effect designates previously married. Likewise, for patient sex, an indicator variable for females could be established taking the value 0 for males and 1 for females.

For each of the N patients in the treated group of interest, a predicted logit is obtained as $y_j = \ln p_j/(1 - p_j)$, where the values of the prognostic variables $(X_{j1}, X_{j2}, \ldots, X_{jk})$ for the jth individual patient are employed in the regression equation (15). The esimate of that patient's probability of encountering the event is then obtained as

$$(16) \quad p_j = \frac{e^{y_j}}{1 + e^{y_j}} = \frac{1}{1 + e^{-y_j}}$$

Under the iterative maximum likelihood procedure $\sum_{j=1}^{N} p_j = A$, where A of the N patients experienced the outcome event.

As an example, Truett et al. (29) employed the logistic regression model to predict the risk of coronary heart disease (CHD) among men as a function of seven risk factors. The coefficients in the regression equation were estimated to be

Equation	Variables
-10.8986	(β_0, intercept)
+ (0.0708)x_1	x_1 = years of age
+ (0.0105)x_2	x_2 = mg/dl serum cholesterol
+ (0.0166)x_3	x_3 = mmHg systolic blood pressure
+ (0.0128)x_4	x_4 = % of ideal body weight
- (0.0837)x_5	x_5 = g/dl hemoglobin
+ (0.361)x_6	$x_6 = \begin{cases} 0 & \text{if never smoked} \\ 1 & \text{if less than 1 pack per day} \\ 2 & \text{if 1 pack per day} \\ 3 & \text{if more than 1 pack per day} \end{cases}$
+ (1.0459)x_7	$x_7 = \begin{cases} 1 & \text{if EGG abnormal} \\ 0 & \text{otherwise} \end{cases}$

Note that the last variable (x_7) is coded as 0 or 1 and is an indicator variable of the type described above. For example, for a man 45 years of age with cholesterol 350 mg/dl, blood pressure 120 mmHg, 160% ideal body weight, hemoglobin 13.0 g/dl, who smokes more than one pack per day and with an abnormal ECG has an estimated logit of risk y = 1.04, with resulting risk of CHD estimated to be p = 0.74.

The Relative Importance of Prognostic Variables

The regression model then can be employed to evaluate the importance of a given prognostic variable, or set of prognostic variables. Although the individual β coefficients and their standard errors are usually obtained, it is generally agreed that the test of the hypothesis that a given coefficient is zero is not always a valid indicator of the importance of a prognostic variable relative to the others in the model. To test the latter, the concept of the addition to sums of squares for regression is employed. This is analogous to the partial F test in multiple regression (see Ref. 31, Chapter 6).

In multiple regression, the total sums of squares (SST) of the dependent variable, $\Sigma(y - \bar{y})^2$, where $\bar{y}$ refers to the mean, is partitioned into two components, one a component due to regression (SSR) and the other error. When the regression model fits the data perfectly, the component of sums of squares due to regression will equal the total sums of squares, i.e., SSR = SST. This results in correlation r = 1, since r^2 = SSR/SST. Further, as additional variables are added to the model, the SSR cannot decrease, and will increase in relation to to the predictive importance of the variables added. Thus, the addition to sums of squares for regression when a variable is added to (or removed from) the model can be used to test the relative importance of that variable relative to those which had already been entered into the model.

For example, consider that a logistic regression model with 10 prognostic variables were employed. The regression model would first be applied to the data based on all 10 variables to yield a χ^2 statistic for regression on 10 df. A model then would be obtained with the first variable removed from the set of predictors to yield a χ^2 statistic on 9 df. The difference in the χ^2 statistics for regression with that variable removed (the equivalent to the addition in sums of squares when that variable is added) can be employed as a χ^2 statistic on 1 df to assess the importance of that variable relative to the others. In like manner, each of the prognostic variables could be considered relative to the others, and the number of variables in the model reduced to a subset in which all variables contained in the model contribute to the overall ability to predict the outcome.

Such a procedure for model building, starting from the full set of prognostic variables, is termed a step-down or backward elimination procedure. Alternately, a step-up or forward selection procedure could be employed in which the one prognostic variable which shows the greatest χ^2 for regression is selected, and then additional prognostic variables added when each in turn produces the greatest increase in χ^2 for regression relative to those already selected. The step-up procedure often requires less computation, but Mantel (32) has shown that a step-down procedure will always identify an optimal subset, whereas a step-up procedure may not.

As with other forms of subgroup analyses, such "model building" also increases the probability of type I error. Given a sufficiently large number of prognostic variables from which to choose, it is highly likely that an optimal subset can be identified by a stepwise procedure, even though in fact those who encounter the event do not differ on any of the prognostic variables in the population at large (see Ref. 33). In building such models, therefore, it has been proposed that at each step variables only be included in the model which show a contribution to regression which is significant with a nominal α level obtained from the Bonferroni inequality Eq. (14) (see Ref. 34).

11.9 REGRESSION ADJUSTMENT OF TREATMENT EFFECTS

A regression model may also be employed to evaluate the differential effects of treatment, adjusting for several prognostic variables in combination. In this case, a set of one or more treatment related variables are added to the model and their contribution to sums of squares for regression is obtained relative to that for the set of prognostic variables, thus providing an adjusted statistical test of treatment differences.

Although an adjustment of treatment effect for the combination of prognostic variables could in principle be conducted using the Mantel-Haenszel procedure, the regression model has the added advantage that continuous prognostic variables can be employed as such in the model, and a much larger number of prognostic variables can be employed in the analysis. On the other hand, the regression model may be highly dependent on the scaling of the treatment indicator or prognostic variables. For example, consider a clinical trial in which a high-dose group (1000 g), a low-dose group (500 g), and placebo group (0 g) are employed. In this case, a variety of treatment indicator variables can be used, including a binary indicator for high dose, a binary indicator for low dose (for placebo both would be 0), actual dose, and various transformations of actual dose. In such cases it is not uncommon to encounter a situation in which no significant treatment effect after adjustment for other variables is obtained using one scaling (such as dose), whereas a significant effect is obtained under some other scaling (such as log dose with 0 for placebo). The use of regression models for treatment adjustment, therefore, should be conducted with caution.

Cornfield (35) was among the first to employ a regression model for the adjustment of treatment effects, although he did not use the addition to sums of squares principle to obtain an adjusted statistical test. Rather, his objective was to obtain an estimate of the proportion of events in the treated group which would have been expected had the composition of the treated group with respect to the prognostic variables been equivalent to that of controls. A logistic model was fit to the data only for the control group to obtain estimates of the β coefficients for each of the prognostic variables. The logistic regression equation then was applied to each of the patients in the treated group to obtain an estimated p_j. The resulting sum of the p_j provided a revised expected number of events for comparison to that actually observed in the treated group. That is, the model provided an estimate of what the control expected event rate would have been had the treated patients received placebo. Alternately, a regression model based on the control group could be applied to the entire study sample to obtain a control-adjusted estimated rate, and a regression model based on the treated group likewise applied to the entire study sample to obtain a treatment adjusted estimated rate, and the two then compared.

Note that this more precise procedure may often yield results different from the application of the regression model based on one group to an "average" patient from another group. In the latter commonly employed procedure, the average values for each prognostic variable within the second group are employed in the regression equation and the resulting p_j interpreted as the average probability of the event for the group as a whole. One should not expect, however, that the expected probability of the "average" patient would equal the average expected probability over the entire group as calculated in Cornfield's procedure.

11.10 LIFE TABLE REGRESSION MODELS

Regression models have also been developed for use with life tables, the most widely employed being the model due to Cox (36), which applies under the assumption of proportional hazard functions among the treated and control groups across time. Under this model the form of the regression equation is

(17) $\lambda(t) = \lambda_0(t) \left[\exp \left(\Sigma_i \beta_i X_i \right) \right]$

where $\lambda_0(t)$ is the hazard function of the underlying survival distribution and $\lambda(t)$ is the hazard function for an individual as modified by the vector of variables, including treatment indicator variables. In life table terminology, the hazard function refers to the attack rate, or simply the proportion of events in an interval, (see Section 9.4). Thus, the Cox model is an extension of the logistic model since

(18) $\ln \dfrac{\lambda(t)}{\lambda_0(t)} = \Sigma_i \beta_i X_i$

The regression coefficients β_i are estimated through an iterative maximum likelihood procedure from which estimated coefficients, standard errors, and an overall χ^2 due to regression are obtained. This model can be employed for predictive analyses or adjustment of treatment effects in the same manner as described above for the logistic regression model. Additional expository articles include Refs. 37 and 38.

11.11 INTERIM STATISTICAL ANALYSES

As described in Sections 7.5, 7.6, and 9.5, it is ethically required that the results of a clinical trial be statistically analyzed as the data accumulate to ensure patient safety and to allow an early termination of the trial if the objectives are met prior to completion of the study. There are basically two statistical approaches to these interim analyses.

Repeated Significance Tests

Interim statistical analyses pose well-recognized statistical problems related to the multiplicity of statistical tests conducted on the accumulating data. These problems have been referred to as sampling to a foregone conclusion (39) or the effects of repeated significance tests (40,41). If the results are examined after each successive block of n observations using a traditional statistical test with significance level

$\alpha = 0.05$ each time, then the true type I error level increases with each successive test (see Section 9.5). An obvious solution, therefore, would be to use a smaller significance level at each successive test so that the true type I error level realized at the end of the study would still be within the desired limits. For example, based on Ref. 40, if 10 successive analyses were to be conducted, each should employ an α level of 0.0107 in order to ensure an overall type I error level of $\alpha = 0.05$ at the conclusion of the study.

Table 11.4 presents the actual α level required for up to 10 repeated tests in order to realize a true type I error $\alpha = 0.05$ or $\alpha = 0.01$ (from Ref. 40). These results are based on successive two-tailed tests using a normally distributed statistic with known variance in which the test is conducted after equal increments in sample size (e.g., after n patients, then 2n, 3n, . . .). In addition to normally distributed statistics, however, these results can be applied to a wide variety of test statistics, including the usual t-test and chi-square test statistics (42). Further, Armitage (43) has developed repeated significance test (RST) sequential plans based on this concept.

TABLE 11.4 Nominal Significance Levels Required for up to 10 Repeated Significance Tests in Order to Realize a True Type I Error Level $\alpha = 0.01$ or 0.05

True α	Number of repeated tests					
	1	2	4	6	8	10
0.05	0.05	0.0296	0.0183	0.0142	0.0120	0.0107
0.01	0.01	0.0056	0.0033	0.0025	0.0021	0.0019

Source: From Ref. 40.

Sequential Analysis

Alternately, many of the statistical procedures for sequential analysis could be applied to the analysis of accumulating data. These sequential procedures (see Ref. 43) are based upon the <u>sequential likelihood ratio</u>, which is calculated after each successive patient has reached an outcome. The sequential likelihood ratio is defined as $\theta = P(x|\mu_0)/P(x|\mu_1)$ where μ_0 specifies the parameter of interest under the null hypothesis of no treatment-control difference, and μ_1 that alternate value of the parameter which reflects the minimal clinically relevant difference which it is desired to detect. The quantity $P(x|\mu)$ refers to the likelihood (e.g., probability) of the observed sample when the hypothesized value of μ is assumed to be true.

In Section 9.5 the concept of likelihood was introduced. In that discussion the <u>area</u> probabilities α and β (type I and type II error) were employed, whereas in the present context likelihood refers to the probability of the exact data value and not the area above (or below) that value. For example, referring to Figure 9.1, $P(x|\mu_0)/P(x|\mu_1)$ would be obtained as the height of the curves for H_0 and H_1, respectively, at the observed value x. The point at which the curves for H_0 and H_1 cross yields $\theta = 1.0$, and for that value of x the two hypotheses are equiprobable. Above this point, $\theta < 1$ indicates evidence in favor of H_1, and below this point $\theta > 1$ in favor of H_0.

As described by Armitage (43), sequential analyses based on θ can be applied to tests of differences in the proportion of events in each group, t-tests of differences in means, and tests of the equivalence of survival curves, among others. The sequential procedure is expressed through the sequential sampling rule $\ell < \theta < u$ where one continues to enter and follow patients so long as $\ell < \theta < u$, where $u = (1 - \beta)/\alpha$ and $\ell = \alpha/(1 - \beta)$, α and β being the desired type I and type II errors. If either sampling rule bound is infringed, the study is stopped, rejecting the null hypothesis H_0 in favor of H_1 as soon as $\theta \leq \ell$, or accepting the null hypothesis if $\theta \geq u$. From this relationship, bounds on the usual test statistic can be obtained after each observation such that the desired type I and type II errors α and β are maintained.

When a two-sided statistical test is conducted, the events $\theta \leq \ell$ and $\theta \geq u$ correspond to the respective conditions that treatment B is better than A or treatment A is better than B. An example is presented in Figure 16.1, which also displays the added feature of truncation, whereby a maximum sample size is also specified. A third boundary is then defined which when reached would lead to acceptance of the null hypothesis of no difference between the therapies.

All the sequential methods based upon this likelihood ratio can also be obtained under a Bayesian procedure in which either or both of the null and alternative hypotheses are specified as intervals rather than a specific point, e.g., H_0 being $a < \mu < b$ for specified values a and b (see Ref. 44).

With a sequential likelihood ratio procedure the accumulating data can be examined repeatedly and the trial stopped as soon as it becomes possible to clearly reject the null hypothesis or to accept it. Further, these procedures have the property that the "stopping rule" incorporates the desired levels of both α and β, and thus ensure that the overall significance level will be limited to the desired level α while the procedure will maintain the desired level of power $(1 - \beta)$.

These sequential procedures, however, are most applicable to clinical trials in which the outcome for each patient is known promptly and in which it is logistically feasible to conduct a sequential analysis as each outcome is observed. Given the logistical problems of data flow and the need for committee review of patient safety, the group sequential methods based upon repeated significance tests are generally preferred.

REFERENCES

1. Sackett, D. L., and Gent M., Controversy in counting and attributing events in clinical trials. N. Engl. J. Med., 1979, 301, 1410-1412.

2. DeMets, D., Friedman, L., and Furberg, C. D., Counting events in clinical trials. N. Engl. J. Med., 1980, 302, 924.

3. Coronary Drug Project Research Group, The Coronary Drug Project: Design, methods and baseline results. Circulation, 1973, 47, 11-150.

4. The Coronary Drug Project Research Group, Clofibrate and niacin in coronary heart disease. J. Amer. Med. Ass., 1975, 231, 360-381.

5. Coronary Drug Project Research Group, The Coronary Drug Project: Initial findings leading to modifications of its research protocol. J. Amer. Med. Ass., 1970, 214, 1303-1313.

6. Coronary Drug Project Research Group, The Coronary Drug Project: Findings leading to further modifications of its protocol with respect to dextrothyroxine. J. Amer. Med. Ass., 1972, 220, 996-1008.

7. Coronary Drug Project Research Group, The Coronary Drug Project: Findings leading to discontinuation of the 2.5-mg/day estrogen group. J. Amer. Med. Ass., 1973, 226, 652-657.

8. Lachin, J. M., Marks, J. W., and Schoenfield, L. J., and the NCGS Protocol Committee and the National Cooperative Gallstone Study Group, Design and methodological considerations in the National Cooperative Gallstone Study: multicenter clinical trial. Controlled Clinical Trials, 1981, 2, 177-230.

9. Schoenfield, L. J., Lachin, J. M., the Steeting Committee, and the National Cooperative Gallstone Study Group, Chenodiol (chenodeoxycholic acid) for dissolution of gallstones: The National Cooperative Gallstone Study: a controlled trial of efficacy and safety. Ann. Intern. Med., 1981, 95, 257-282.

10. Mantel, N., and Haenszel, W., Statistical aspects of the analysis of data from retrospective studies of disease. J. Nat. Cancer Inst., 1959, 22, 719-748.

11. Mantel, N., Chi-square tests with one degree of freedom: extensions of the Mantel-Haenszel procedure. J. Amer. Statist. Ass., 1963, 58, 690-700.

12. Fleiss, J. L., Statistical Methods for Rates and Proportions, Wiley, New York, 1973.

13. Miettinen, O., Estimability and estimation in case-referent studies. Amer. J. Epidemiol., 1976, 103, 226-235.

14. Fleiss, J., Confidence intervals for the odds ratio in case-control studies: The state of the art. J. Chron. Dis., 1979, 32, 69-77.

15. Cornfield, J., A statistical problem arising from retrospective studies., in Proc. 3rd Berkeley Symp. on Mathem. Statist. and Prob. (J. Neyman, ed.), University of California Press, Berkeley, Calif., 1956, pp. 135-148.

16. Mantel, N., and Fleiss, J., Minimum expected cell size requirements for the Mantel-Haenszel one-degree-of-freedom chi-square test and a related rapid procedure. Amer. J. Epidemiol., 1980, 112, 129-134.

17. Birch, M. W., The detection of partial association, I: The 2 x 2 case. J. R. Statist. Soc., B, 1964, 26, 313-324.

18. Landis, J. R., Heyman, E. R., and Koch, G. G., Average partial association in three-way contingency tables: A review and discussiuon of alternative tests. Int. Stat. Rev., 1978, 46, 237-254.

19. Zelen M., The analyses of several 2 x 2 contingency tables. Biometrika, 1971, 58, 129-137.

20. Halperin, M., Ware, J. H., Byar, D. P., Mantel, N., Brown, C. C., Koziol, J., Gail, M., and Green, S. B., Testing for interaction in an I x J x K contingency table. Biometrika, 1977, 64, 271-275.

21. Mantel, N., Brown, C., and Byar, D. P., Tests for homogeneity of effect in an epidemiologic investigation. Amer. J. Epidemiol., 1977, 106, 125-129.

22. Bishop, Y., Feinberg, S., and Holland, P., Discrete Multivariate Analysis: Theory and Practice, MIT Press, Cambridge, Mass., 1975.

23. Cutler, S. J., and Ederer, F., Maximum utilization of the life table method in analyzing survival. J. Chron. Dis., 1958, 8, 699-712.

24. Kaplan, E. L., and Meier, P., Nonparametric estimation from incomplete observations. J. Amer. Statist. Ass., 1958, 53, 457-481.

25. Mantel, N., Evaluation of survival data and two new rank order statistics arising in its consideration. Cancer Chemother Rep., 1966, 50, 163-170.

26. Peto, R., Pike, M. C., Armitage, P., Breslow, N. E., Cox, D. R., Howard, S. V., Mantel, N., McPherson, K., Peto, J., and Smith, P. G., Design and analysis of randomized clinical trials requiring prolonged observation of each patient: II. Analysis and examples. Brit. J. Cancer, 1977, 35, 1-39.

27. Peto, R., and Pike, M. C., Conservatism of the approximation $\Sigma(O-E)^2/E$ in the log rank test for survival data or tumor incidence data. Biometrics, 1973, 29, 579-584.

28. Miller, R., Simultaneous Statistical Inference, McGraw Hill, New York, 1966.

29. Truett, J., Cornfield, J., and Kannel, W., A Multivariate analysis of the risk of coronary heart disease in Framingham. J. Chron. Dis., 1967, 20, 511-524.

30. Lachenbruch, P. A., Discriminant Analysis, Hafner Press, New York, 1975.
31. Draper, N. R., and Smith, H., Applied Regression Analysis, Wiley, New York, 1966.
32. Mantel, N., Why step-down procedures in variable selection. Technometrics, 1970, 12, 621-625.
33. Lachin, J. M., and Schachter, J., On stepwise discriminant analyses applied to physiologic data. Psychophysiology, 1974, 11, 703-709.
34. Kupper, L. L., Stewart, J. R., and Williams, K. A., A note on controlling significance levels in stepwise regression. Amer. J. Epidemiol., 1976, 103, 13-15.
35. Cornfield, J., The University Group Diabetes Program: A further statistical analysis of the mortality findings. J. Amer. Med. Ass., 1971, 217, 1676-1687.
36. Cox, D. R., Regression models and life tables J. Roy. Statist. Soc., B, 1972, 34, 187-220.
37. Breslow, N. W., Analysis of survival data under the proportional hazards model. Int. Stat. Rev., 1975, 43, 45-58.
38. Prentice, R. L., and Kalbfleisch, J. D., Hazard rate models with covariates. Biometrics, 1979, 35, 25-39.
39. Cornfield, J., Sequential trials, sequential analysis and the likelihood principle. The Amer. Statist., 1966, 20, 18-23.
40. Armitage, P., McPherson, C. K., and Rowe, B. C., Repeated significance tests on accumulating data. J. Roy. Statist. Soc., A, 1969, 132, 235-244.
41. McPherson, K., Statistics: the problem of examining accumulating data more than once. N. Engl. J. Med., 1975, 290, 501-502.
42. Pocock, S. J., Group sequential methods in the design and analysis of clinical trials. Biometrika, 1977, 64, 191-199.
43. Armitage, P., Sequential Medical Trials, Wiley, New York, 1975.
44. Lachin, J. M., Sequential clinical trials for normal variates using composite hypotheses. Biometrics, 1981, 37, 87-102.

12
The Crossover Design

AVIVA PETRIE*
London School of Hygiene and Tropical Medicine
and Royal Postgraduate Medical School
London, England

12.1 INTRODUCTION

The presentation thus far has focused on the simple group comparison trial, which is the most prevalent in clinical research. In this design each patient receives either the experimental or control therapy. An often employed alternative design is the crossover trial, so called because each patient receives both treatment and control, or vice versa, in succession, i.e., crosses over from one therapy to the other. Thus each patient serves as his own control.

    The crossover design is most applicable when there is considerable between-patient variability and less within-patient variability. The crossover design can only be used when there are short-term changes due to therapy which reverse rapidly. It is particularly useful in chronic disease because the state of the disease must be as severe at the second administration as at the first administration. This in turn requires that there be a withdrawal interval between the first and second

---

*Ms. Petrie is currently with the London School of Hygiene and Tropical Medicine, London, England.

administration of sufficient duration for the effects of therapy to completely dissipate.

If these conditions are met, the crossover design can be a powerful tool because each patient contributes twice as much data as in the simple group comparison and fewer patients may be needed. For example, if one wished to have a sample size of 50 per group, i.e., 50 periods of active treatment and 50 periods of control therapy, a total of 100 patients would be randomized under a group comparison design (50 to each group), whereas only 50 patients would be required in a crossover design as displayed in Figure 12.1.

Although the crossover design is commonly used, it is most frequently employed in the assessment of a pharmacological effect, such as a serum assay, rather than the longer term clinical effects, such as healed versus not healed. Thus, the crossover design is frequently used in the preclinical evaluation of a new drug which precedes the assessment of clinical efficacy or toxicity.

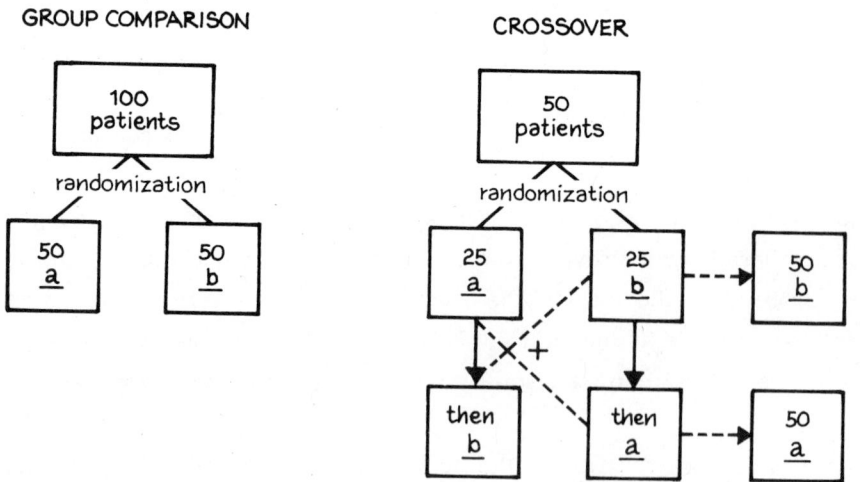

FIGURE 12.1 The crossover design and the group comparison design compared, each with 50 patients receiving treatment a and 50 patients receiving treatment b.

The technique is as follows: For the comparison of two treatments, an active and a control therapy, each patient receives both the active treatment and the control therapy. Because the order of administration may be important, as may be the time of administration, the order in which each patient receives the active treatment and the control therapy is assigned at random. If the active treatment and the control therapy are called a and b, respectively, some patients receive a followed by b, and the remaining patients receive b followed by a. The sequence assigned to each patient, a-b or b-a, is determined by randomization.

A typical design is as follows:

Start (t_0): Randomization of a patient to sequence a-b or b-a. Start first administration (a or b).
One month (t_1): End first administration. Begin withdrawal interval.
Two months (t_2): Start second administration (b or a).
Three months (t_3): End second administration.

The patient's condition is then assessed at each of the four time points, the start and end of each administration. Usually continuous measurements are employed, such as serum cholesterol levels (mg/dl), and the data are analyzed using analysis of variance techniques.

The methods for the proper analysis and interpretation of the results of a crossover design are presented by Grizzle (1) and others (2-4). Briefly, the most important requirement is that there be no carry-over effects from the first administration to the second. This is most easily tested by examining the mean change $t_2 - t_0$ for the patients in the a-b sequence compared to that for the patients in the b-a sequence.

As an illustration, the results of a hypothetical crossover trial are presented in Figure 12.2. The carry-over effects of the administration of drug in the first period are clearly evident and thus invalidate any conclusion drawn from data obtained in the second administration period. In this case there would be no recourse but to analyze only the

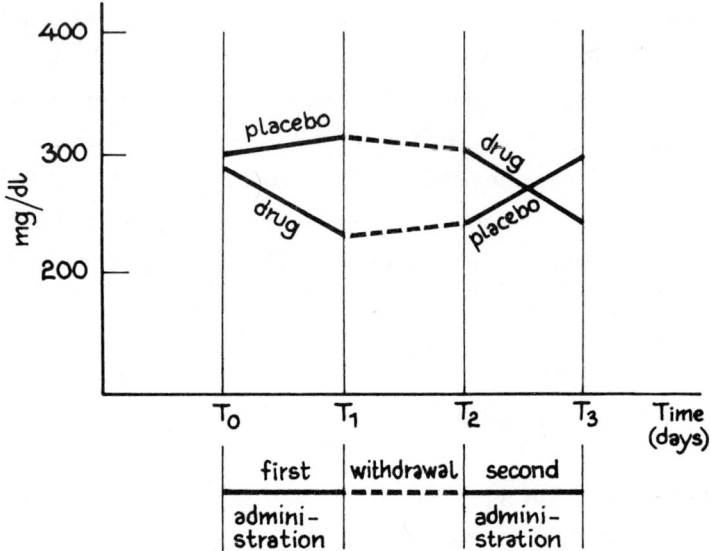

FIGURE 12.2 Mean serum cholesterol levels (mg/dl) for patients assigned to receive placebo then drug, and those assigned to receive drug then placebo, in a hypothetical crossover trial.

data obtained from the first period of administration as though it were a simple group comparison trial.

12.2 DISCUSSION

Ingelfinger
If the only limiting factor, philosophically, is that the condition being tested, the disease, the abnormality, has to be of approximately equal severity at the start of the two periods, I wonder why there are not more trials of this type. Certainly it requires fewer patients than the usual two-group trial.

Riis
The problem of carry-over effects is a major obstacle to the use of this method.

Schoenfield
The requirements for this design are an agent which produces a rapid and relatively transient response, that is, a response that comes and then goes relatively rapidly; and a steady-state physiological condition,

an unchanging disease, during the period of observation. It is also very important in this type of design that every patient completes the study. Loss of a patient during the trial might jeopardize the validity of the study. These requirements should be recognized when considering the use of this design. In summary, I think a crossover design is useful, particularly when a limited number of patients is a problem, and particularly with considerations of the limitations of the design.

Chalmers
I think it is good that we realize there are a wide variety of designs that could be employed. In my experience I have used a good many of them, including the crossover. I am convinced, however, that the best approach overall is to use the simplest design possible, unless it is absolutely necessary, unless there is no other way to achieve the objectives of the study.

Ingelfinger
But what is the simplest design? The simplest design that we all use in medicine, uncontrolled, is to try different treatments in the same patient. That is the basis of conventional clinical management. Therefore, I would argue that the simplest design is the crossover. We do not have to worry about having a comparable patient, it is a 50 year old male who smoked during the whole time; many of the variables are intrinsically controlled. The only variable that has really remained steady is the disease state.

Chalmers
The crossover, however, is different from ordinary clinical management in that the time when the therapy is administered or withdrawn is predefined and not based on how well the patient responds.

For example, we were once asked to evaluate a patient because he was thought to show that bedrest is essential in treating hepatitis. When originally admitted to the hospital, he had an elevated bilirubin and was put to bed. It came down. After it came down he got up and his bilirubin went up again. So he was put to bed and his bilirubin came down again, and he got up and his bilirubin went up again. This clearly proves that bedrest cures jaundice in hepatitis, and ambulation makes it worse. When the patient was transferred to us, we put him to bed or let him up at random, and the bilirubin elevations had no relation to bed rest.

Doctors are constantly falling into this trap. When they plan to give the patient a treatment, they wait to start it until he is worse, they wait to stop it until he is better, they start it again if he relapses, and they conclude because of the obvious time relationship that the treatment caused the changes. This is not true of the crossover design.

Tygstrup
I think that the general agreement is that the crossover design should be treated very carefully, and that in most situations it should be avoided.

REFERENCES

1. Grizzle, J. E., The two-period change-over design and its use in clinical trials. Biometrics, 1965, 21, 467-480, (Corrigenda, 1974, 30, 727.)
2. Koch, G. G., The use of nonparametric methods in the statistical analysis of the two-period change-over design. Biometrics, 1972, 28, 578-584.
3. Cochran, W. G., and Cox, G. M., Experimental Designs. Wiley, New York, 1968.
4. Snedecor, G. W., and Cochran, W. G., Statistical Methods, The Iowa State University Press, 1967, Ames, Iowa.

Part IV
Implementation of the Randomized Clinical Trial

13
Elements of an Ideal Protocol

LESLIE J. SCHOENFIELD
Cedars-Sinai Medical Center
University of California at Los Angeles
Los Angeles, California

13.1 INTRODUCTION

The preceding chapters have reviewed the clinical and statistical considerations in the design, execution, and analysis of a clinical trial. This and subsequent chapters review the implementation of a clinical trial, starting with the considerations in writing a study protocol.

There are eight basic elements which should be considered in the development of the protocol for a study (Figure 13.1). Each of these elements interrelate to produce the final product, a workable protocol.

The Introduction

The introduction to the protocol presents the background scientific information that provoked the determination that there is a need for the study. The introduction brings the field up to date and clarifies the state of the art. It provides what is currently known about the natural history of and therapy for the disease, and the mechanism of action, efficacy, and safety of the proposed treatment. From this emerges a statement of the rationale from which the critical hypothesis is developed.

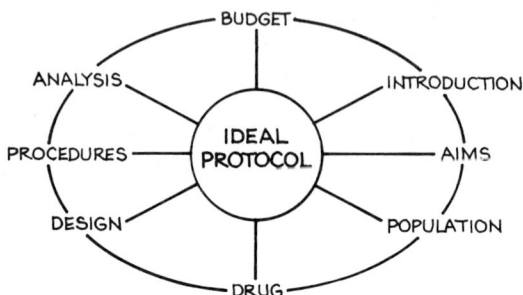

FIGURE 13.1 The interrelationships between the elements of an ideal protocol.

A statement to be used to obtain informed consent then follows from this review of the known or suspected risks and potential benefits of the experimental therapy and the natural history of the disease. Guidelines for experimentation with human subjects are described later in Chapter 19, but it should be mentioned that the mechanism of informed consent and its contents are included in the development of the protocol.

Aims and Objectives

The introduction usually is followed by the statement of the aims, which should be based directly on the hypothesis to be tested. A decision must be made as to whether the protocol aims describe a long-term or short-term study. As has been emphasized previously, the aims must be stated simply and concisely. Furthermore, the aims should be realistic in relation to the available facilities, patient population, and resources, and be applicable to the specific hypothesis that is to be tested.

Study Population

The next requirement is a precise description of the patient population and the disease under study. The critical predetermination of sample size has been discussed at some length in Chapter 9. The recruitment and accession of patients are also major concerns, even at this stage.

Thus, an integral consideration in the determination of sample size is a realistic assessment of the potential rate at which patients will actually enter the study. This depends on the characteristics of the available base population, the catchment area, labor, facilities, recruitment efforts of the treatment centers, and the requirements of the protocol.

Eligibility and exclusion requirements have already been discussed in Chapters 4 and 5. It is at this stage that the eligibility and exclusion criteria for the study population are precisely defined. This includes a clear and precise definition of the disease state and its stage of severity in the patients under study.

In preparing these sections of the protocol the dilemma of a balance between eligibility and exclusion must be resolved. Restrictive eligibility criteria may create an irrelevant study population, whereas broad criteria engender uncontrollable factors. There are also implications for sample size requirements, since prognostic heterogeneity will increase sample size requirements, whereas prognostic homogeneity may restrict the patient "pool" from which study subjects may be recruited.

Experimental Drug or Procedure

The fourth element of the protocol is a description of the experimental drug or procedure to be evaluated. In a drug trial the purity specifications and chemical and physiological characteristics of the drug, including bioavailability and shelf life, are pertinent. For example, a study could be invalidated if the agent loses potency during the latter part of the experiment. Similarly, the drug must be absorbed predictably and efficiently and be available without major loss through its metabolism or interactions with other drugs. Accordingly, the appropriate formulation, dose, route, and schedule of administration of the drug must be specified.

Compliance also requires consideration. Studies of compliance in clinical practice and in experimental programs have shown that perhaps as many as 30% of patients may not ingest the prescribed agent according to the specified schedule (1). Special efforts to stimulate patient motivation, therefore, are necessary to improve compliance. The ideal procedure would be to use an inert marker or signal within the drug to indicate to the investigators whether each patient is complying. The development of optimally efficient, precise, and practical inert markers, however, has not yet been accomplished.

Likewise, the specifications for the control therapy must be developed. If a placebo control therapy is to be employed, the placebo should be an inactive agent which looks, feels, weighs, smells, and even tastes the same as the active agent. Patients often taste the contents of capsules in an attempt to determine whether they are receiving the active ingredient or a placebo. Thus, the formulation of an appropriate placebo requires careful planning and the consultation of a clinical pharmacologist could prove helpful.

If a study is designed to assess two agents with distinctly different appearances, for example, azathioprine, prednisone, both, or placebo, in the treatment of chronic active hepatitis, then a double-dummy placebo technique can be adopted. A placebo is prepared for each agent. Each patient participating in the study receives two different "medications." Thus, patients in the azathioprine group receive azathioprine and the placebo for prednisone; those in the prednisone group receive prednisone and the placebo for azathioprine; those in the combined group receive both prednisone and azathioprine; and those in the placebo group receive both placebos.

Experimental Design

The statement of the experimental design includes the rationale for the sample size determination, the follow-up schedule to be employed, and the design features to be implemented. These issues have been discussed extensively, but it should be remembered that the essential considerations are randomization, controls, and blinding. It is at this stage that any ethical, scientific, and statistical conflicts must be resolved. For example, if an agent is potentially hepatotoxic, under which conditions (if any) should liver biopsy with its attendant risks be performed, and how often? In addition, the logistical, budgetary, and administrative aspects of the study may influence the selection of an experimental design.

Procedures and Methods

The sixth component of the protocol is the specification of the procedures and methods. Implementing the protocol, especially the preparation of the procedures manual and forms in a multicenter trial, and its pretesting will be discussed in Chapter 15. At this stage of protocol preparation, however, the various procedures must be specified for the evaluation of each outcome (e.g., efficacy and safety), for clinical management, and for ancillary research. The procedures for the diagnosis and treatment of intercurrent illness, management of potential toxic effects of the agent, and manifestations of the disease under study all should be predetermined. Uniform techniques are essential for all procedures, and the observations must be made at prescribed intervals which should not be changed during the study.

For all procedures, both internal and external quality control helps assure reproducible data with known reliability and validity. Unreliable data or unvalidated measurement techniques obviously negate the value of a carefully chosen and executed experimental design. A note of caution, however, should be inserted regarding the potential expense of quality control procedures.

Analysis

Given the above, the methods of statistical analysis to be employed should readily be specifiable. The types and frequency of analyses should be predetermined, recognizing that both interim and final analyses are usually necessary. Moreover, the outcome criteria for efficacy and safety, including the definitions of dropouts, withdrawals, treatment success, and treatment failure, should be established at this stage. In fact, the contents of the anticipated published manuscript should be considered; thinking about a tough editor should prompt scrupulous attention to the details of the protocol.

Facilities and Budget

Finally, the protocol should realistically consider the necessary and available facilities and the projected budget. If the available facilities will be taxed by the protocol requirements, then a multicenter organization might be considered; or if the budget is excessive, then it may be necessary to reevaluate all the other protocol elements, starting with the aims. Often one goes through the complete process a number of times before a final protocol evolves.

Each of the components of the protocol should then be developed, tested, and reworked before implementing the study. Protocol changes during a study can produce bias, unreliable results, and grief.

REFERENCE

1. Sackett, D. L., Magnitude of compliance and uncompliance, in Compliance with Therapeutic Regimens (D. L. Sackett and R. B. Haynes, eds.), Johns Hopkins Press, Baltimore, Md., 1975, pp. 9-25.

14
Achieving an Adequate Sample Size: The Multicenter Trial

NIELS TYGSTRUP
Rigshospitalet
University of Copenhagen
Copenhagen, Denmark

Whenever a clinical trial is conducted, the result should be highly conclusive whether it is a positive or negative result; that is, there should be a small type I and type II error, a small α and β. The trial should also usually be able to detect a small difference between the treatments, a clinically relevant difference. The combined effect of these objectives will be to increase the required sample size; therefore, it may be necessary to seek ways to increase the sample size. Two important determinants of sample size are the study duration (time) and the size of the population base from which patients can be drawn.

14.1 STUDY DURATION

Study duration may be employed in either (or both) of two ways to increase sample size. The first is to lengthen the period of patient recruitment, thus allowing a longer period within which more patients can be accrued. If 50 patients per year can be recruited, then the sample size can be increased by simply lengthening the period of recruitment.

Study duration may also be adjusted to increase the period of follow-up of patients. This is most beneficial when there is a common closing date follow-up period (see Chapter 7) and the outcome event of interest occurs rather evenly over time; i.e., the event rate is not zero beyond a certain point. This is most applicable in studies of long-term mortality, such as due to myocardial infarction, and less applicable to studies of morbidity of chronic diseases.

For example, in a study of the healing rates of duodenal ulcer, little benefit would be reached by extending the follow-up period, since the healing rate beyond 12 weeks could be expected to approach zero. On the other hand, consider a study of mortality in which exponential survival applies. As shown in Chapter 9, the sample size and study duration are based on a fixed number of deaths being required, say, 100 deaths for a particular study. If the study were to last only 5 years, then 200 patients might be required to yield the 100 deaths or 40 patients per year. For such a study it might be easier to extend the period of follow-up to reduce the numbers of patients needed each year.

There is a limit, however, to the use of time as a means of increasing the sample size, in terms of either total numbers of patients or total numbers of patient months of follow-up. Treatments tend to have a limited lifetime, the average half-life estimated to be 10 years. If a large fraction of this period is used to conduct a trial, there may be no interest in the results when they finally appear.

Therapies are subject to development as well as to fashion, and a decrease in interest will result in a fall in the referral rate to the trial. Figure 14.1 shows the cumulative growth of a cooperative European trial on corticoid treatment in fulminant liver failure. After 3 years the curve tends to flatten, possibly because the participating investigators lost interest in the study, not because patients weren't available.

Somehow, most doctors feel it a burden to collect data for a clinical trial, but good data are only produced by persons motivated for the trial. Most data collectors are trainees. Trainees spend a limited time in the same unit, and so cannot expect to see the results--or their name among the list of authors in the report. Their motivation will

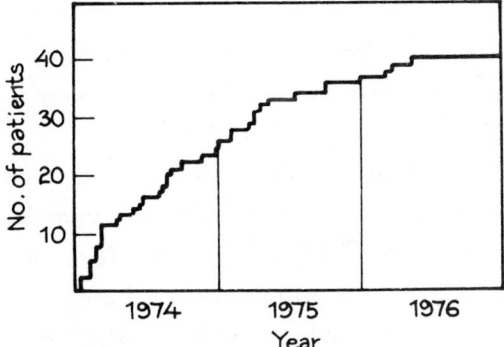

FIGURE 14.1 Cumulative number of patients recruited by 17 centers into the Acute Liver Failure Trial of the European Association for the Study of the Liver.

deteriorate, and thus also the quality of the data they collect. Poor data will decrease the signal-to-noise ratio, and as a result, the minimal detectable difference will increase with time instead of decrease, as expected.

It is difficult to see exactly when this happens, but it is a rule of thumb that trials should be conducted, if possible, in less than 3 years.

14.2 THE MULTICENTER TRIAL

Often the only means of obtaining the required sample size is to increase the population base from which the sample can be drawn by organizing a multicenter study. However, there is no simple proportionality between the geographical area included, the benefits in terms of statistical power, and the ability to detect a clinically relevant difference. Geographical variation of diseases and the prevalence of prognostic factors may contribute to variability, which may bring noise into the data. Likewise, there is geographical variation among physicians, differences in education and background which may mean that they use different diagnostic criteria and evaluate treatments in a different way. Furthermore, distance may affect motivation. The further the participating unit is from the center responsible for the trial, the more difficult it may be to make the unit adhere devotedly to the protocol.

The way to reduce the deteriorating effect of time and distance on the multicenter trial is to prepare for it with these problems in mind. The protocol of a multicenter trial has to be very specific regarding criteria of selection and exclusion, rules for withdrawals and dropouts, treatment schedules, follow-up studies, and outcomes. The large amount of preparation necessary then adds to the cost and overall duration of multicenter trials.

However, there are also benefits to be obtained. First, a very specific protocol in general will give more reliable and reproducible results than will a casual one, simply because variability in medicine is so great that unless great efforts are made to reduce it, it will obscure the results. Second, data collected from many different areas will provide information about geographical variation which may be of great interest from an epidemiologic viewpoint. Third, the results obtained in a trial covering a wide geographical area may be more useful than those from a trial depending on a very narrow population, because there will be greater confidence in the wide applicability of the results.

There is one additional effect of international multicenter trials which I think deserves recognition. They may stimulate international standardization of diagnostic criteria and methodology, and on the whole promote international cooperation and understanding, which in my view is a merit in itself. When such trials become more common, these advantages will increase, and hopefully the costs will be reduced as more experience is obtained and routine procedures developed.

14.3 DISCUSSION

Selecting Cooperating Investigators in the Multicenter Trial

Riis

Many departments may be interested in joining a trial, but at the end one finds that only a few have provided most of the patients. The main reason is that most departments lack deep motivation and knowledge of the study protocol.

Lachin
One of the important problems in multicenter trials is that a physician who is not ethically prepared to conduct the study may want to jump on the bandwagon. A physician should not participate in a clinical trial unless he is convinced that it is ethically appropriate to randomize, unless without hesitation he would be willing to assign any patient to either of the alternative therapies. A physician who is not ethically prepared may in fact undermine the trial by failing to accrue his share of the patients, or if biased against the treatment, by only entering patients with poor prognosis.

Schoenfield
I feel that the selection of participating centers in a multicenter trial should be conducted objectively. The initial step should involve some form of advertisement to the clinical research community that a multicenter trial is about to begin. The potential participants should know the requirements to be expected of the treatment centers, and they should be asked to submit a proposal as to how they would participate. The proposals should demonstrate an understanding of the aims and of the methods of the particular trial. Preferably, the centers participating in a multicenter trial should have some experience in controlled trials, not necessarily multicenter trials.

The individuals running the center should have expertise in the area studied, but often the established investigator is very busy and it may be difficult for him to give the appropriate time to the study. Thus, the key individuals participating within each treatment center should also be identified.

In this way, it is possible to make objective decisions about the potential contributions of the applicants to participate in the multicenter trial.

Wright
In a multicenter trial on non-Hodgkins lymphoma we tried to maintain interest by finding physicians who had a research interest in the patients entering the trial. For example, some investigators were interested in the immunology of lymphoma, and therefore, although they were not the clinicians who were involved, they still tried to recruit patients into the trial for their own studies.

Authorship Citation in the Multicenter Trial

Chalmers
There is another aspect of multicenter trials which has to do with motivation. A successful cooperating unit depends on a young investigator to do all the hard work. That person is devoting half or more of his time for 1, 2, or more years to make the study work. If the

study reports are then written and published by a multicenter study group, that person has lost years of his life as far as his bibliography is concerned.

The clinic investigator needs to have recognition as one of the major contributors to the study. That is why a multicenter trial should be reported by all the investigators, no matter how many they may be. The journal article should list all the participants as authors so that each investigator can include the report in his bibliography as a paper to which he contributed.

Some journals have settled this by putting the investigators in a footnote. I maintain that it takes no less space to put it in the masthead. Editors need to be convinced that the success of a cooperative trial depends on the young investigator and that he can be expected to do a better job if he gets credit for it in his bibliography.

Ingelfinger
The editor's point of view is a matter of practical and esthetic nature. Suppose there are 40 authors and they are listed in the conventional way, that is, in larger type than the text, not in small footnote type. When the reader opens a journal he sees the title, then he has to skip past a whole page and maybe the next page of authors. Then finally the text begins. I think this is absurd. Furthermore, it is a financial question affecting publication severely. Every extra page costs $900 to $1000 in a large circulating journal. We cannot afford to waste space for all these names. That is why journals like the footnote idea with the small print. But it is also true that if the authors' names are put in the footnote they will not be listed as authors in the Index Medicus.

ADDITIONAL READINGS

Croke, G., Recruitment for the National Cooperative Gallstone Study. Clin. Phar. Ther., 1979, 25, 691-694.

Prout, T. E., Perceptions of the coordinating center: As viewed by the principal investigators. Controlled Clinical Trials, 1980, 1, 127-141.

15
The Execution of a Protocol

JOHN M. LACHIN
The George Washington University
Washington, D.C.

This chapter reviews the various considerations in the execution of a protocol, and I shall do so from the perspective of a multicenter cooperative clinical trial. All these considerations also apply to the single-investigator trial as well, though obviously on a smaller scale.

As a starting point, it must be emphasized that the most important consideration in making any trial a success is to start with a realistic protocol. Many studies are doomed to failure before they actually begin because the protocol is simply unrealistic. For example, a protocol that winds up with a small sample size due to poor initial projections of patient availability, and has power less than 50%, is a waste of time.

15.1 ORGANIZATION

Given the protocol specifications, an organization should then be developed which is sufficient to assure that the protocol is properly and efficiently implemented. To demonstrate what this entails, consider the organization developed for the National Cooperative Gallstone Study (NCGS), as shown in Figure 15.1 from Ref. 1. There is a steering

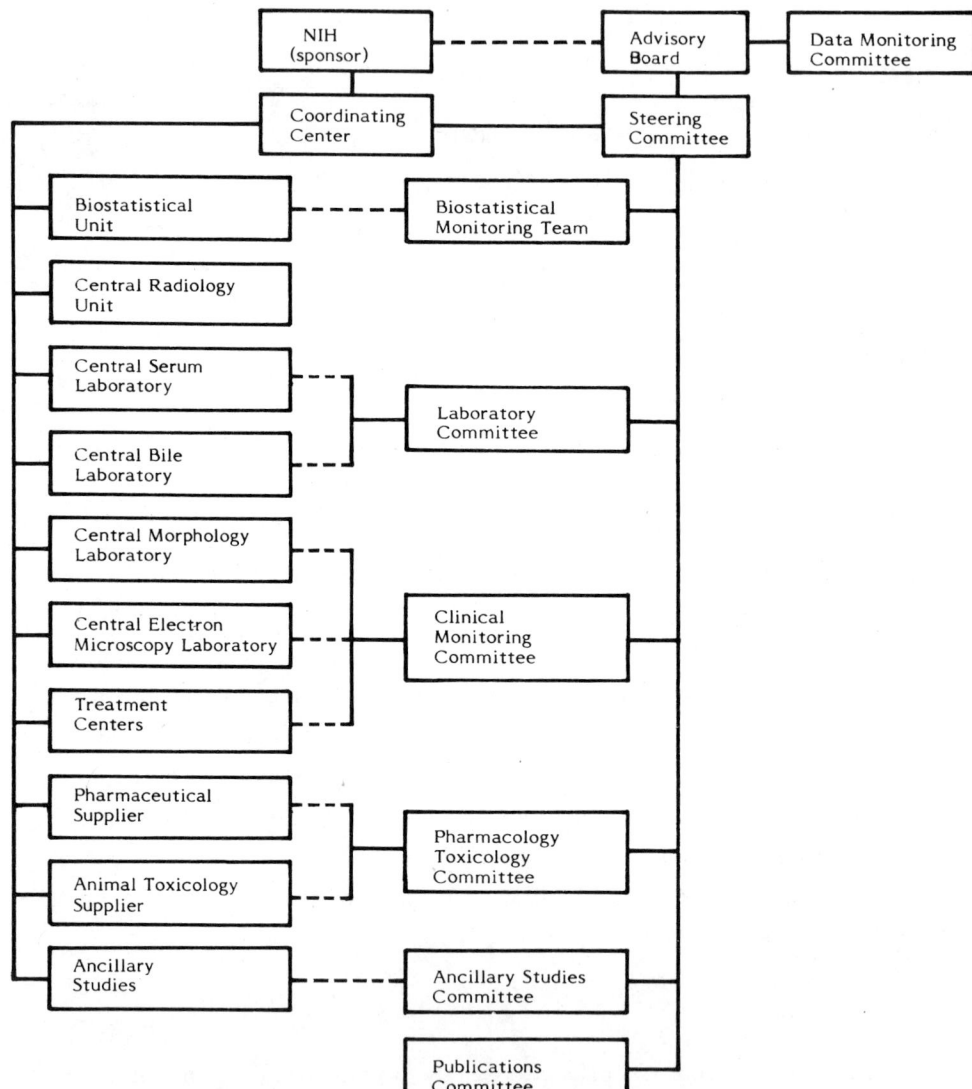

FIGURE 15.1 Organizational structure of the National Cooperative Gallstone Study (NCGS). (From Ref. 1.)

committee of scientists responsible for the overall scientific integrity of the study. They meet regularly to review all activities in the study and its overall progress. The coordinating center is the administrative arm of the steering committee and administrates the day-to-day execution of the study. The <u>biostatistical unit</u> is responsible for all design considerations, randomization, the collection of the data, and its analysis. In this study the biostatistical unit is separate from, though administratively part of, the coordinating center. In many cooperative studies both functions are housed in a single unit.

The <u>advisory board</u> oversees the functions of the steering committee and the coordinating center, and considers issues of ethics and policy. The <u>data-monitoring committee</u> is a group of investigators, both physicians and statisticians, who are not involved in the study in any way, and who review the data as they are collected in order to assess efficacy and safety (risk-benefit). In many studies, the functions of the data-monitoring committee are assumed by the advisory board. Recall that it is ethically demanded that interim analyses be conducted as the data are collected, and the National Institutes of Health has adopted a guideline for the establishment of a data-safety monitoring committee for all NIH-sponsored clinical trials, which is presented in Appendix A. Thus, the primary responsibility of the data-monitoring committee is to recommend protocol changes based on the emerging results in order to protect the welfare of the study patients while maintaining the integrity of the study.

The <u>clinical monitoring committee</u> consists of physicians who review all the procedures for clinical management used in the study. A clinical monitoring committee is very important in a study in which the project physicians make decisions about dosage levels and withdrawal from treatment or perform subjective evaluations of treatment outcome. Many studies have been biased because the physicians have not managed all patients in a uniform manner, and this is especially a distinct possibility in any study which does not have a double blind. The mere presence of a clinical monitor which provides peer review of clinical decisions helps to prevent this.

There are many other organizational units specific to this study, but the above are the major organizational components. Of importance to any clinical trial is that the study be organized according to the separate activities necessary to ensure the success of the trial. The NCGS chose to do this through the use of committees, whereas for a small trial these roles could be fulfilled by individuals.

15.2 STANDARDIZATION

The next thing necessary is to standardize all the protocol procedures. This is true not only of a multicenter trial, but even a single-center trial in which there are two or more physicians treating patients, two or more technicians, and so on. It must be specified beforehand exactly how everything is to be done. The slightest error in procedures, the slightest variation, can have drastic consequences on the conclusions.

Usually these specifications are delineated in a separate procedures manual or manual of operations which is more detailed than the study protocol. This document must be very extensive in order to ensure the success of the study. For example, consider the chapter headings to the NCGS Procedures Manual as presented in Table 15.1. The manual describes policy matters, such as informed consent, the evaluation of treatment center performance, and the mechanism for protocol changes. It specifies patient recruitment procedures; eligibility and exclusion criteria; how the study medications are labeled, distributed, and randomly assigned; the procedures for dosage level adjustments; and the schedule and description of visit procedures. It specifies standardized clinical management procedures for all expected clinical situations possibly related to the treatment or the disease. It specifies the exact manner in which all procedures are to be conducted, from drawing a blood sample to conducting a liver biopsy. Everything that is to be done in the trial is specified in detail beforehand, including outcomes, statistical analyses, and how the data will be published.

15.3 STUDY FORMS

Accompanying the procedures manual is the development of the study forms, i.e., the documents used to collect information from the study.

TABLE 15.1 NCGS Procedures Manual Table of Contents

Part I: Introduction

    1. Background and development
    2. Objectives and study design
    3. Organization
    4. Policy matters
    5. Patient recruitment

Part II: Evaluation and follow-up

    6. Patient eligibility and exclusion criteria
    7. Randomization and drug packaging
    8. Drug administration
    9. Dosage level adjustment
   10. Schedule and description of patient visits
   11. Dropouts and withdrawals
   12. Management of illness
   13. Permanent cessation of therapy

Part III: Procedures

   14. Radiological procedures
   15. Determination of gallstone volume and number
   16. Procedures for duodenal intubation
   17. Procedures for liver biopsies
   18. Procedures for electrocardiogram
   19. Collection and handling of laboratory specimens
   20. Laboratory evaluations and tests
   21. Medication procurement and handling
   22. Treatment center procedures

Part IV: Data handling and analysis

   23. Completion and mailing of forms
   24. Data management procedures
   25. Endpoints and statistical analyses
   26. Publicity and publications

Supplements

    A. Protocol of the initial study of hepatic morphology
    B. External quality control procedures

In a large study these forms will be computerized and used as the basis for all analyses. The forms should be developed with the following issues in mind.

1. The study forms should be <u>standardized</u>. The information needed to evaluate the objectives should be obtained from all participants in an identical manner.
2. The questions on a form should have <u>construct validity</u>; they should measure what they are intended to measure. Each item must be very carefully worded. If the purpose of a question is to obtain a past history of biliary tract surgery, it should not ask for a history of abdominal surgery; otherwise, hysterectomies and cholecystectomies will be recorded under the same item and tabulated together.
3. A related concept is that every form should be <u>coherent</u>. The items should be organized in a logical manner, and the meaning of every item should be very clear.
4. The forms should be <u>thorough</u>. They should include all the information the statistician and the physician require to evaluate the objectives of the study. They should include all the major outcomes and any other necessary information.
5. The forms should be <u>streamlined</u>. They should not contain auxillary information that is irrelevant to an evaluation of the objectives. Information needed by the physician for the routine management of a patient may not be needed to evaluate the objectives and thus should not be incorporated into the standardized study forms. This is clearly an important but also difficult process.
6. The forms should be based on the trial's <u>activities</u>; that is, there should be a separate form for each prinicpal activity to be conducted. Data from a pathology report should not be collected on the same sheet of paper used to collect data from a history or

Execution of a Protocol   225

a physical examination. These sets of information come from two different sources, and if it is all to be recorded on one form, that form may get lost in the transfer, although this is less important in a small single-center trial.

Of course, there should be detailed instructions on forms completion, either as a separate document, or incorporated directly into the forms through comments.

15.4 COMPUTERIZATION

Since virtually all analyses will likely be conducted via computer, consideration should be given to computerization and data management. This process begins with forms design. Some of the additional considerations are the following:

1. Each study form type should have a distinct identification number (e.g., form 1, form 2).
2. Each form type should employ a standardized section to record patient and visit identification.
3. Fill-in-the-blank items should be avoided in preference for precisely directed questions. For example, rather than

    Describe any symptoms present: _____
    _____

    the following would be preferable:

    Is the patient experiencing any of the following symptoms?
    Diarrhea   No ( )   Yes ( )
    Nausea   No ( )   Yes ( )
    and so on

4. For numerical items, the exact number of digits and units of measurement should be specified. For example

    Body weight: __ __ __ . __ kg

Since the study forms will be the basis for later statistical analysis, their proper construction is crucial.

The development of a <u>data management system</u> to process accumulating data by computer is beyond the scope of this presentation. An adequate data management system, however, should afford the following basic capabilities for

1. Editing of key data items for errors, i.e., missing data, out of range (e.g., body weight above 200 kg), or internal inconsistencies (e.g., male with five pregnancies)
2. Updating a computerized data record to correct errors
3. Internal auditing to ensure that all forms received are properly accounted for at each stage of processing
4. Back-up of all study files to protect against a disaster, such as a fire in the computer center
5. Inventory of all data received for each patient
6. Extraction of key data items from the computerized study files for statistical analysis

All these elements (forms design, forms computerization, and data management) culminate in the final statistical analyses, and the validity of these statistical results is highly related to the extent to which these prior steps were executed adequately.

15.5 TRAINING AND PRETESTING

Once the above are accomplished, perhaps the most crucial step in ensuring that the trial mechanism will work is to properly train all personnel and then pretest all procedures and forms in order to get the bugs out. Due to their complexity, clinical trials are invariably subject to Murphy's law: if anything can possibly go wrong, it will.

Since the majority of the errors will occur in the early stages of the study, a <u>pilot period</u> is usually required during which training and pretesting proceed concurrently. Of course, a formal pilot study is not always possible, although this is by far the best approach. Some trials have employed instead the concept of pilot patients, who are simply the first patients treated and who act as an advance guard. Other studies have used a certification procedure, whereby treatment center personnel are trained, tested, and then certified by the study through examinations. Personnel are then allowed to participate in the study only after certification. The issue, however, is not how one trains personnel and pretests procedures, but simply that they be done.

15.6 QUALITY ASSESSMENT

Once the trial starts, a mechanism should be established for the ongoing assessment of the quality of the trial procedures. Every process should be checked continually to make sure that the procedures are being followed properly.

1. The recruitment process should be monitored to ensure that recruitment proceeds at a steady pace. If the treatment centers recruit patients too quickly, the patient visits may pile up later and the staff may not be able to both handle all the return visits and maintain additional recruitment. In most cases, however, just the opposite problem arises--recruitment lags. In this case, continual monitoring of the rate of recruitment and the reasons patients are being excluded from each center may lead to a more effective recruitment program.

2. The evaluation for eligibility should be monitored for each incoming patient. There is usually a sound reason for all selection criteria, and the randomization of an ineligible patient benefits neither the study nor the patient. Some studies have been critized or doubted because large numbers of ineligible patients were entered who were at risk for, and who later developed,

complications. Their presence thus greatly confuses the analysis and interpretation of the results.

3. The <u>randomization process</u> should be monitored to make sure there is no breaking of the code, to make sure that patients are properly randomized and that the blinding is being preserved. The sample composition should be monitored as patients are being recruited to detect any inadequacy in the statement of the eligibility criteria.

4. The <u>conduct of all procedrues</u> should be monitored. There should be external quality control surveillance for laboratories as described below.

5. The <u>collected data</u> should be continually monitored to ensure that forms are properly completed, that forms are completed when they should be, that each patient's visits occur when they should. If the protocol specifies follow-up visits every 6 months, that does not mean every 4 months or every 9 months.

6. Finally, the <u>data analysis</u> should be monitored, checked, and rechecked. It should be done twice in different ways to make sure there are no computational errors.

All the above will require additional mechanisms and procedures to provide these built-in checks. On the most basic level, reports on the performance of each study unit may prove adequate to detect gross inadequacies in procedures, e.g. forms submitted with errors, improperly labeled laboratory specimens, and overdue patient visits. Such reports will identify the presence of problems but not always their cause. Thus, it is usually necessary to periodically site-visit each operational study unit to review problems and procedures. This is mandatory in a multicenter trial and is always enlightening.

The most effective means of quality assessment, however, are the procedures for <u>external quality control surviellance</u>, which are usually employed to assess the performance of laboratories, e.g., serum, but are equally applicable to any measurement procedure. In the laboratory setting this entails the blind analysis of two basic types of quality control samples

1. <u>Known standards</u>, e.g., a serum sample drawn from a large pool with a stable and known constitutent level
2. <u>Split duplicates</u>, e.g., a second aliquot of serum drawn from the same vial as a prior aliquot analyzed in a prior batch

Known standards allow one to assess long term drift and the <u>accuracy</u> of the measurements during the life of the study, and the analysis of a group of such results provides an assessment of the <u>validity</u> (see Chapter 10) of the measurement methodology within the range of values provided by the standard. Thus, it is usually preferable that two or more standards be employed, such as serum standards with a high and low constituent level.

Split duplicates allow the assessment of the <u>precision</u> of the measurements, and analysis of a group of such paired results (original result and split-duplicate result) provides an assessment of the <u>reliability</u> (see Chapter 10) of the measurement methodology.

One or more of the above mechanisms can be used for ongoing quality assessment of all study procedures and units, and their implementation should be carefully considered in any clinical trial.

15.7 MORALE

Finally, the morale of study personnel should be considered. A study is only as good as the physicians, the affiliated staff, and the patients incorporated into it. They all must maintain an acute interest in and dedication to the success of the study. Physicians should be kept informed of the study's development as much as possible without unblinding or biasing their evaluations. The affiliated staff are always an important consideration, for they are often the most important members of the study team. The clinic coordinator who schedules patient visits, who talks with the patients before they see the doctor, can have an enormous effect on the study. The individuals who record the data on the study forms and handle laboratory specimens can have a greater impact on the success or failure of the trial than the physician who treats the patients. Finally, the patient is always the foremost consideration in the conduct of any clinical trial. If the patient ever feels he is not being treated in what we consider to be his best interest, we are both losing.

15.8 DISCUSSION
Organization

Schoenfield
Figure 15.1 presents the extensive organization of the National Cooperative Gallstone Study, with each block in this particular instance standing for a committee or unit or group of physicians and scientists. But that need not necessarily be so. This is a very complex multicenter study. An army is not necessarily needed to conduct a clinical trial. The point to be emphasized is that all these functions or activities should be considered by the investigators, but the function of the advisory board can be served by an individual, that of the clinical monitoring committee by an individual, and so on.

Riis
The normal protocol is dealing with a rather small trial in one department. The forms will cover 10 to 12 pages at most, and perhaps two to four doctors will participate, and they of course will serve all these functions themselves. All the functions mentioned should still be served, but it is much easier.

Study Forms

Petrie
I would like to comment on the record form which is the information sheet that is filled in with details about the patient and then passed on to the statistician. The statistician then computerizes the information and analyzes it from the computer. It is important, therefore, that the information be transferred correctly from the record form to the computer. If the actual data are quantified, then the information will be entered into the computer as it comes off the information sheet in quantitative terms. Otherwise, if it is qualitative, then a code must be devised so that it can be put in numerical terms in the computer. Since we want as few mistakes as possible, the record forms should be designed with this in mind.

There are a number of ways of capturing the desired information. One way involves having someone read the physician's records and coding the data onto a transfer sheet. The data are then keyed into the computer from the transfer sheet. Thus there are three stages of information transfer, one from the physician-patient interview to the physician's records, one from these records to the transfer sheet, and one from the transfer sheet to the computer. But every transfer stage is liable to introduce mistakes. Thus, if possible, the transfer sheet should be done away with and the forms designed so they can be used as the primary source documents to enter the data directly into the computer. This of course will require that every item of data be precoded on the record form. This will have the added advantage of standardizing the physician-patient interview to ensure that all the desired questions are asked by all participating physicians of all patients, hopefully in the same way.

Pilot Studies

Wright
I would ask the panel if they have any observations on the importance of a pilot study?

Riis
By a pilot study I assume you mean an initial small study of 10 or 20 patients according to the protocol of the full-scale trial. In this case, the pilot study is a pretest of how the real trial is going to work physically and operationally, but nothing more. I do not think that trends in the pilot study should be examined in hopes of seeing results that would save having to do the full-scale trial.

Chalmers
In general, I think that the pilot trial is a great danger, especially the uncontrolled pilot trial. Randomization should take place with the first patient, for two reasons. First, in the pilot trial, experience is needed with the placebo or the control patient just as experience is needed with the therapeutic patient. Second, if randomization is not included with the first patient, the pilot trial may very likely be misleading because patients may be selected such that there is no way to avoid looking at the results. If the ideal patient is selected, he is going to have an ideal result, and then there arises an ethical dilemma. How can I do a randomized trial when I am now convinced by the pilot trial that the new therapy is superb? On the other hand, if I selected very sick patients who deteriorate, then I become convinced by the pilot trial that the therapy is no good, and therefore I don't do the randomized trial. So I think a major reason for the shortage of controlled trials is the fact that people started with uncontrolled pilot studies and decided that they could go no further. They then go ahead and publish the pilot trial.

A <u>randomized</u> pilot trial is different, however, since it blends in with the final trial without any reason to exclude its patients from the final analysis, and in this case I feel it can be helpful.

Ingelfinger

There is an important difference between these two kinds of pilot trials. Dr. Riis recommends a pilot in which the techniques of the proposed randomized controlled trial are being tried out to see if they work without any regard to the effect of the treatment on the patients. Dr. Chalmers agrees but denounces the pilot trial in which the investigator includes an attempt to see how the treatment works. Now, the facts are, at least in the United States, that many people disagree with Dr. Chalmers' view. It is my impression that most investigators feel that they should carry out a pilot trial with emphasis on the effects of the drug.

Chalmers

I feel the heart of the issue is that the uncontrolled pilot trial has serious ethical problems. Let me use an example. Suppose a surgeon has developed a new operation. I urge him to randomize the first patient but he refuses and goes ahead and operates on a series of patients because he says that he has to develop the operation before he can compare it with the standard operation. He says that if he did compare both operations from the beginning his new operation would look bad because he was just working it out. In fact, suppose he is right and it would have looked bad because 8 of the first 12 patients died. He then says he was right not to have done a randomized pilot trial.

To me this epitomizes the ethical reason why he had to do a randomized pilot trial. What he did was to subject the first patients to a high death rate in order to develop a new technique. He should have been honest to the patient and said, "I'm going to use a new surgical technique and I am unwilling to randomize you because at the present I think it is worse than the standard procedure." Obviously, he could not get informed consent because if he had asked for informed consent, the patients would have said, "Thank you very much, but I will have the standard operation. Try it out on somebody else.

He could, however, have approached the patient by saying, "I have not yet perfected this operation in man. It may be worse, it may be better. I would like your permission to be randomized, and if you end up with the standard operation and it proves to be better you will be better off. If you end up with the new operation and it proves to be better you will be better off there. Either way you have a 50% chance of getting the better therapy."

It is always ethically more acceptable to obtain informed consent; the only truly informed consent that can be obtained to try a new operation or a new drug, is if randomization is built in.

Wright
I find myself in disagreement with the rest of the panel. I think there are different types of pilot studies. I agree that it might be said that randomization should be employed immediately, but the alternative is to look at the effects of the drug and on the basis of clinical experience to determine whether the controlled trial is going to be useful. After a pilot, the investigator is not convinced of the drug's worth, but he is assessing the possibility.

Chalmers
I disagree, because if the pilot trial results are accepted, positive or negative, then afterward how can patients be randomized? Patient consent to randomization can only honestly be obtained if it is not known whether the new therapy is going to be effective.

Lachin
It has been said that the pilot study can give results that would allow making a decision to go ahead with the main trial. If the pilot is also randomized, there are a variety of "two-stage" statistical procedures which could be employed to analyze the data in this fashion (2,3). The problem, however, is that most pilot studies are not formally conducted this way and have a small sample size. What, then, if the results are negative? Is the trial stopped, realizing that power may only be 30%, realizing that there may be very severe selection biases? I agree with Drs. Riis and Chalmers. The only real function of a pilot study should be to get the bugs out of the procedures, and it also should be randomized.

Petrie
One last reason for using a pilot study is to estimate the degree of variation to be observed in the measurements. This may be valuable in determining the sample size needed for the complete trial.

Riis
I think that editors could help greatly to clean up the field if they would simply not allow pilot studies to be published. Every time a pilot study with its trends is published I think the field is polluted. I agree that we have to do small studies in the beginning, but I also think we should be obliged to go on with a controlled trial before publishing.

REFERENCES

1. Lachin, J. M., Marks, J. W., and Schoenfield, L. J., and the NCGS Protocol Committee and the National Cooperative Gallstone Study Group, Design and methodological considerations in the National Cooperative Gallstone Study: A multicenter clinical trial. Controlled Clinical Trials, 1981, $\underline{2}$, 177-230.

2. Day, N. E., Two-stage designs for clinical trials. Biometrics, 1969, $\underline{25}$, 111-118.

3. Colton, T., and McPherson, K., Two-stage plans compared with fixed-sample-size and Wald SPRT plans. J. Amer. Stat. Ass., 1976, 71, 80-86.

ADDITIONAL READINGS

Coronary Drug Project Research Group. The Coronary Drug Project: Design, methods and baseline results. Circulation, 1973, 47, 11-150.

Ederer, F., Practical problems in collaborative clinical trials. Amer. J. Epidemiol., 1975, 102, 111-118.

Fredrickson, D. S., The field trial; some thoughts on the indispensable ordeal. Bull. N.Y. Acad. Med., 1968, 44, 985-993.

Greenberg, B., Conduct of cooperative field and clinical trials. American Statistician, 1959, 13, 13-17.

Grizzle, J. E., The case for management research for large field trials. J. Chron. Dis., 1977 30, 257-259.

Lachin, J. M., Prout, T. E., Overton, H. H., Rifkind, B. M., Berge, K. G., and Sedransk, N., Perceptions of the coordinating center. Controlled Clinical Trials, 1980, 1, 125-152.

16
Early Termination of a Clinical Trial

THOMAS C. CHALMERS
The Mount Sinai Medical Center
Mount Sinai School of Medicine
New York, New York

16.1 THE DECISION TO STOP

Whether to terminate a clinical trial while in progress requires a process which is a constant mixture of three different disciplines: biostatistics, ethics, and clinical practice. If the decision is reached that the study should be stopped at a certain point, it should be based not only on the fact that the data will be clinically meaningful, but also on considerations that they are biostatistically valid and ethically acceptable.

The last point is the most complicated and difficult because it involves a consideration not only of the ethical responsibility of the physician for the welfare of the individual patients who are already in the study and will continue in the study, but also the welfare of the patients who might later be enrolled into the study, and perhaps most important the welfare of all other patients with that disease for whom the therapy might be indicated. Thus, consideration must also be given to the extent to which a study might be continued for the good of patients not in the study but who will develop or have the disease in the future. This in turn depends on the degree of threat or danger or disadvantage to the patients in the study. In other words, if the patient loses nothing by staying in, a study might be continued until it is more valid biostatistically.

On the other hand, if the welfare of the patients in or about to come into a study might be compromised by continuing, and if the conclusion is becoming fairly certain but is not biostatistically "significant," then there is an extremely serious ethical problem. Even informed consent is not sufficient to warrant continuing the study according to some standards. Thus, we can imagine a decision point moving back and forth to varying degrees within a triangle along the dimensions of clinical relevance, biostatistical validity, and ethical propriety.

It is absolutely crucial, therefore, that every protocol have a section prepared in advance which considers the clinical, ethical, and biostatistical aspects of how the study is to be terminated. One has to evaluate the relative advantages of a fixed sample size without looking, a fixed sample size with frequent looks and what that does to the α level, and formal methods of sequential analysis. Sequential analysis is something we all talk about but I have the feeling it is a little like the crossover design. It looks neat, it sounds neat, but it is practically never used formally.

16.2 ADDITIONAL CONSIDERATIONS

In addition to stopping, one must also consider modifying factors, considerations which may lead to a change in the experimental design because of something that has happened during the study. For instance, if a study is designed to evaluate whether an assumed safe therapeutic agent is helpful in a given disease, there is no justification for continuing the study to prove beyond any doubt that it is harmful, even though a trend in that direction has barely reached significance.

A good example is the University Group Diabetes Program (UGDP) (1). The UGDP is the most disputed and I think the most valuable, superb, correct, authentic trial ever conducted. The UGDP was stopped when the p-value was about 0.02 for excess mortality among those treated with an oral hypoglycemic agent (depending on the type of analysis it was between 0.01 and 0.05). Those who wanted to continue using the drug have criticized the UGDP investigators for not continuing the study long enough to prove beyond a shadow of a doubt (i.e. $p = 0.01$ or less) that a drug which was supposed to be helpful was really killing people. This is entirely invalid.

One could have argued that if there had not been so much prior belief in the efficacy of the medicine, they should have stopped with a p-value of 0.2, instead of 0.01, because there was no evidence that the drug was doing any good, at least as far as the original aim of the study, to determine whether the drug reduced the cardiovasular complications of diabetes. Thus, if the direction of the trend is opposite from that which may be beneficial, the study should be stopped sooner.

Another modifying factor is the dropout rate. If the dropout rate becomes so large that there is no point in continuing the study because it will no longer be statistically valid, it should be stopped and a new design attempted which would not result in such a high proportion of dropouts. This is especially true if the dropout rate is differentially distributed, so that, for example, more of the placebo group is dropping out than the therapeutic group.

The most informative clinical trial I ever conducted was one of the efficacy of ascorbic acid in the prevention of the common cold, which was carried out among employees of the National Institutes of Health (2). We recognized that it would be hard to get people to take two capsules of ascorbic acid three times a day for 12 months; so the protocol specified that the study would be stopped if the dropout rate reached 30%. It was determined that 200 subjects were needed to provide the desired power, and thus 300 patients were recruited to allow for a 30% dropout rate. The protocol also specified that if the dropout rate was significantly greater in the placebo group, the study would be stopped, and this in fact occurred. With a p-value of 0.2 more people on the placebo were dropping out than on the ascorbic acid. It turned out that these doctors and nurses were opening the capsules and tasting them, and could tell the difference between ascorbic acid and placebo. Those who found they were on placebo dropped out as soon as they had a cold; whereas those who were on ascorbic acid stayed in, and that's why the study was stopped. The study was continued long enough, however, to show there was no evidence whatever that ascorbic acid prevented colds, and that there was a significant shortening of the colds only among those who admitted tasting the capsules. Among those who guessed wrongly or did not admit tasting the capsules, the duration of the colds was identical. So it was a botched-up study; we stopped but learned a lot from it.

16.3 BLINDING

Among the most important, and perhaps the most controversial items of all, are the importance of blinding the trends, and the importance of having all decisions about stopping as well as protocol modifications being made by one or more physicians and statisticians who have no stake in the study. The important decisions should be made by scientists and clinicians who have no personal involvement, who are not taking care of patients in the study, who did not write the protocol, who are not dependent on the budget or the funds for their living, and whose reputation is not involved in the study.

I feel this is absolutely necessary, because the physician who is admitting a patient to a clinical trial has a primary responsibility to that patient and not to the trial. We have to accept that when a physician persuades himself and a patient that a trial is good for that patient, he does so because he does not know which therapy is better, and because the patient has a 50% chance with randomization that he will receive whatever treatment will turn out to be better. As soon as the project physician feels that one therapy is superior, his ethical

Early Termination of a Clinical Trial 239

participation cannot be maintained, even though the data are inconclusive. Thus, the project physician should be blinded to emerging results and these decisions left to uninvolved, objective scientists.

A hypothetical sequential trial is presented in Figure 16.1. The patients are admitted in matched pairs and randomly assigned to treatments A and B. If the treatment B patient is better than the A patient in each pair then the line moves down, and when A is better than B it moves up. Let us assume that we have reached the point where we only need one more pair to prove that treatment A is better than treatment B as shown in Figure 16.1. It is still possible, a 6% chance, that the line will reverse and later cross the line of no difference, but there is a 94% chance that the trial will end with A declared better than B.

Let's make it dramatic and assume that this is a surgical trial with the outcome operative mortality, and only a few more patients are needed to finish the study. Do we have the right to ask the next two

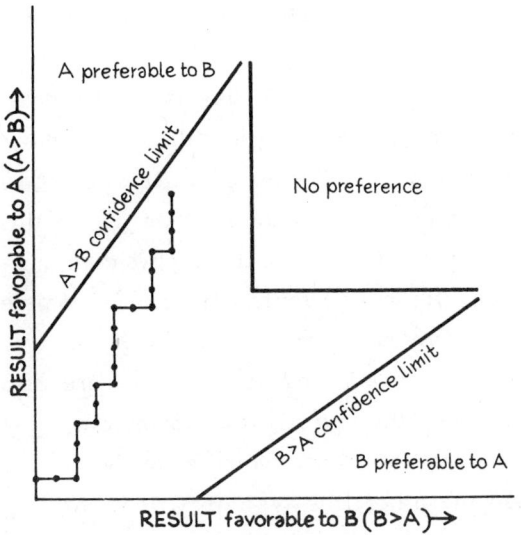

FIGURE 16.1 Sequential analysis of a hypothetical randomized clinical trial.

patients to enter a study in which we know that the chances are highly probable that the one that gets treatment B will die and the one who gets treatment A will survive? This really epitomizes the terrible ethical problem for which there is no easy solution. The only answer I know of, unless we are to say that all clinical trials are unethical, is to say that when the physician enters the patient into the study it has to be with the prior agreement among them that the physician taking care of the patient will not know the trends, and that another objective group will make the decision about when the study should be stopped.

The reason this is critical is that it is a meaningful problem from the very beginning of the trial. We assume before we start that it is equally likely that A or B is better. Now assume that the first pair shows B to be better. The evidence now favors B over A; the chances are very slim, 0.5001 versus 0.4999, but they are there. If the physician knows that the patient who got better had received B, he can no longer, after the first pair, look the patient in his eyes and say the chances are equal that he will do well on either therapy. So it is because of this that I think we must blind the physician and investigators to preliminary data.

I call this the <u>Harkness dilemma.</u> A layman (Harkness) demonstrated this phenomenon to me one evening in a discussion about the ethics of randomization and I became convinced. It is a moral dilemma with no precise answer and so we do the best we can in this moral world. The reason we have to do this is that the physician must prescribe the best known therapy for his patients. He can randomize only if he does not know which therapy is better.

In addition to the medical-ethical justifications, there are also strong statistical reasons for blinding the investigators to the emerging results. If the investigator is aware of trends which strongly suggest that one therapy is better than the other, the type of patient entering the study may change with the progress of the study. Once the physician has realized that one therapy may be better, he often finds some reason, perhaps unconsciously, not to randomize patients with a unique opportunity to benefit from one of the therapies, and they might then get that therapy ex cathedra, out of the study. The physician may then let in the patient who is sicker or to whom the therapy will make no difference, and thus the efficacy of the therapies under study is blunted with time. Thus, there are not only ethical reasons for keeping the results from the investigators, there also are scientific reasons.

16.4 DISCUSSION
The Ethical Dilemma

<u>Student</u>
If there is such an ethical dilemma with a sequential trial, is there also an ethical problem with the fixed sample size trial?

<u>Chalmers</u>
I used sequential analysis only because this is an easy way of illustrating the problem. Suppose a fixed sample size had been agreed on and only one more patient was needed to complete the final number, but this last patient might be assigned to the therapy which up to that point is the worst. Isn't there more of an ethical problem in deciding to admit that patient if he might receive a therapy which is almost proven to be bad? He is going to be used to prove it is bad. Should he not be offered the opportunity of informed consent? Suppose he was told that this study was being done, that the trend now showed it was almost certain that one treatment was bad, but he was needed to enter the study and get that bad treatment in order to prove it was bad. How many people do you think you could get to enter the study? Yet this is what we mean by informed consent. We mean we are telling the patient the benefits and risks when entering a study. So I know no solution to the dilemma other than that there could be a trend but the treating physician doesn't know it.

<u>Lachin</u>
I would like to present a real life example as an illustration of the dilemma. Table 16.1 presents the results of a sequential trial of acute leukemia in which the outcome of interest was mortality (3). These results were used by Schneiderman in a discussion of when this trial should be stopped (4). Again matched pairs were employed, and each patient was randomized to receive therapy A or B. For every patient pair either A or B was better, and let's assume that everyone knew the results as they occurred.

When a group of physicians are shown these results line by line and asked when they would have felt ethically compelled to stop the study,

TABLE 16.1 Outcome of a Sequential Trial on Acute Leukemia

Preferred treatment		Preferred treatment	
Patient pair	Choice	Patient pair	Choice
1	A	11	A
2	B	12	A
3	A	13	A
4	A	14	B
5	A	15	A
6	B	16	A
7	A	17	A
8	A	18	A
9	A	19	A
10	A	20	A
		21	A

Source: Reprinted by permission from Freireich et al. The effect of 6-mercaptopurine on the duration of steroid-induced remissions in acute leukemia, Blood, 1963, 21, 699-716, Grune & Stratton.

usually few would be willing to go beyond the twelfth pair. The fact is, however, that the trial did not reach statistical significance (at the 0.05 level) until the eighteenth pair. The remaining pairs had been randomized at this point but not yet completed their evaluations.

Ingelfinger
I think it is very important to distinguish between trying something new which might be harmful, and establishing whether something which is in universal practice is actually harmful. In the latter case I don't think the emerging results should be examined at all. The trial should be continued right through because there then is an ethical responsibility to provide results that will be as convincing as possible to the medical community in order to stop the abuse of an established technique or drug which is actually harmful.

Chalmers
But then you are thinking of the good of the whole at the sacrifice of the individuals in the trial.

Lachin
One never knows what to expect in a clinical trial. For this reason I think it is very important that the data be examined as they emerge, whether the study involves an established agent or a new agent. The UGDP is a beautiful example of this; the increase in cardiovascular mortality was contrary to all prior expectation even though it was a study of established agents.

Blinding the Results

Blum
I would like to get some practical advice. Suppose there is a study in which two types of operations are being compared. Naturally this cannot be a double-blind study and everybody in a clinic knows there is a trend in favor of one operation after a period of time. How could such a trial be blinded?

Chalmers
This is one of the advantages of a cooperative study. The data would be gathered in multiple institutions, and when one institution has one operation better while the others might have the other better, no single institution knows what the total is.

Lachin
But it would still affect the behavior within an institution.

Schoenfield
I think Dr. Blum's question is really very critical to the whole area of surgery, and I feel there are satisfactory techniques for this type of evaluation. Suppose there is a monitor to determine the eligibility of the patients coming into the study. Having decided that a patient can undergo either one of the two operations being tested, the patient is entered into the study and randomized. Let's say an ulcer operation is being studied. At random, patients are either assigned to undergo vagotomy and pyloroplastic or to undergo enterectomy and vagotomy. A team of surgeons capable of doing either operation then performs the assigned operation on the patient and then will no longer see that patient. Another team could then evaluate the patient's outcome while not knowing which operation the patient received.

Blum
This could be done, theoretically, but I think the surgeon who does an operation will want to know what happened. I have never known a surgeon who did not also care for the patient in the direct postoperative period.

Schoenfield

The internist cares as much for his patient that he gives a medication to, no less than a surgeon who operates. What we need are two teams that have confidence in each other. If I am going to turn my patient over to a colleague, I know he will do whatever is proper for the patient according to the protocol, and I do not have to worry about that.

Play the Winner Rules

Blum

Rather than usual randomization with sequential analysis, why couldn't many studies be conducted according to play-the-winner rules (5)?

Lachin

The best explanation of the "play-the-winner rule" is the example of playing two slot machines in a casino. Suppose one of the slot machines pays off more frequently and we will win more times with this than the other machine. We don't know which one is the better machine, so we randomly pick one and crank the first time. If we win we crank the machine again, if we lose we switch to the other one. Every time we win we stick with that machine. As soon as we lose we switch to the other machine.

This is the most basic form of the class of adaptive allocation schemes whereby the processes of treatment assignment and data monitoring are combined (6). The idea is that sooner or later the better therapy (the winning machine) can be identified with a good deal of confidence while at the same time having maximized the number of patients to receive the better treatment (our earnings) during the trial. This is not a randomized design, and only one outcome is evaluated, not all the other outcomes that might be relevant. Play-the-winner rules have been one of the major arguments used against randomization (7), but these procedures have a variety of deficiencies (8).

Chalmers

The reason that I don't like the play-the-winner rule is that it destroys the blindness critical for adequate randomization. When a patient is accepted for a study, the physician should never have an inkling there is more or less than a 50% chance of which therapy that patient will be assigned to. If a study is done on a play-the-winner basis, the physician knows what therapy the next patient is going to receive, and then all his biases can influence the choice of who gets into the study and who stays out. I don't think the biostatisticians who advocate play-the-winner rules appeciate how easy it is for a clinician to allow his bias to reject or accept a patient for a study.

Tygstrup

The procedure is also limited in that it can only be used if each patient has an immediate reaction to the therapy in only one outcome of relevance. If a delayed reaction is expected, it is difficult to apply because the outcome of the last patient should be known in order to determine how the next patient is to be treated.

Chalmers
For these reasons, I have never seen these methods used. I have only seen them advocated.

After the Trial Is Stopped

Lachin
I would like to make another point about the issue of stopping. Suppose we are dealing with survival curves, and after 3 years of follow-up we decide to stop the study. In doing so we should keep in mind that it is just 3 years of follow-up, how do we know that in the long run the survival curves might not reverse themselves? It is possible that at an intermediate point the curves are statistically significant, but a reversal is still possible. Thus, in deciding to stop a trial, one must also consider whether such a reversal is possible and the probability of its occurrence.

Schoenfield
This raises another type of problem. Suppose we are evaluating the efficacy and safety of a new drug and after 3 years of follow-up the treatment is found to be more effective and safer than the control, at that point in time. Therefore, the treatment is indicated. My question now is: How do we treat the control patients? Suppose this agent caused cancer 5 years later; how would we know if we now gave the treatment to the controls? But on the other hand, how could we not give treatment to the controls since we have just shown the treatment to be effective and safe?

Chalmers
But you haven't shown that it doesn't cause cancer in 8 years.

Schoenfield
That is the dilemma. There is no easy answer, but I think one might resolve this by considering the study aims. When designing the protocol one has to clearly state the aims in terms of short-term or long-term goals. Short term may be a few weeks or a few years, depending on the disease studied and the aims.

REFERENCES

1. University Group Diabetes Program, A study of the effects of hypoglycemic agents on vascular complications in patients with adult-onset diabetes. Diabetes, 1970, 19, 1-830.

2. Karlowski, T. R., Chalmers, T. C., Frankel, L. D., Kapikian, A. Z., Lewis, T. L. and Lynch, J. M., Ascorbic acid for the common cold: A prophylactic and therapeutic trial. J. Amer. Med. Ass., 1975, 231, 1038-1042.

3. Freireich, E. J., Gehan, E., Frei, E., Schroeder, L. R., Wolman, I. J., Anbari, R., Burgert, E. O., Mills, S. D., Pinkel, D., Selawry, O. S., Moon, J. H., Gendel, B. R., Spurr, C. L., Storrs, R., Hauriani, F., Hoogstraten, B., and Lee, S., The effect of 6-mercaptopurine on the duration of steroid-induced remissions in acute leukemia. Blood, 1963, 21, 699-716.

4. Cutler, S. J., Greenhouse, S. W., Cornfield, J., and Schneiderman, M. A., The role of hypothesis testing in clinical trials. J. Chron. Dis., 1966, 19, 857-882.

5. Zelen, M., The play-the-winner rule and the controlled clinical trial. J. Amer. Stat. Ass., 1969, 64, 134-146.

6. Simon, R., Adaptive treatment assignment methods and clinical trials. Biometrics, 1977, 33, 743-749.

7. Weinstein, M. C., Allocation of subjects in medical experiments. N. Engl. J. Med., 1974, 291, 1278-1285.

8. Byar, D. P., Simon, R. M., Friedewald, W. T., Schlesselman, J. J., DeMets, D. L., Ellenberg, J. H., Gail, M. H., and Ware, J. H., Randomized clinical trials--perspectives on some recent ideas. N. Engl. J. Med., 1976, 295, 74-80.

ADDITIONAL READINGS

Chalmers, T. C., Randomized clinical trials in surgery, in Controversy in Surgery (R. L. Varco and J. P. Delaney, eds.), W. B. Saunders, Philadelphia, Pa., 1976, pp. 3-11.

Klimt, C. R., and Canner, P. L., Terminating a long term clinical trial. Clin. Pharmacol. Ther., 1979, 25, 641-646.

Meier, P., Terminating a clinical trial--the ethical problem. Clin. Pharmacol. Ther., 1979, 25, 633-640.

Pocock, S. J., Size of cancer trials and stopping rules. Brit. J. Cancer, 1978, 38, 757-766.

Part V
Perceptions of the Randomized Clinical Trial

17
Randomized Clinical Trials and the Producers

LESLIE J. SCHOENFIELD
Cedars-Sinai Medical Center
University of California at Los Angeles
Los Angeles, California

What are the techniques whereby a clinical trial can be made attractive to the producers, in this context, the physicians and their staff who conduct the trial? The essence of the answer to this question lies in the motivation and morale of the personnel at the participating centers. Are they happy and eager to conduct the trial? Although at first glance this question seems most relevant to a multicenter trial, this also pertains to a single-center trial.

17.1 SELECTION OF PARTICIPANTS

A major consideration relates to the selection of participating clinical centers. In Chapters 13 and 14 we discussed the factors that pertain in the selection of clinical centers; these include the size of the patient population, encatchment area, a track record in clinical trials, and support of the local institution. The selected investigators should have appropriate background and experience, and thereby have a special interest in the conduct of the trial. They need not, however, be internationally recognized experts who may not have sufficient time to devote to the trial.

Once selected, the physicians at each of the clinical centers should be given the opportunity to participate in the development of the protocol. This fosters a sense of contribution, loyalty, and confidence. Furthermore, unique problems at the different treatment centers can be confronted and solved during formulation of a workable protocol. Also, the general informed consent form benefits from the requirements and input of the individual clinical centers.

All this will help ensure that the requirements of the protocol are realistic. The types of observation, the forms, and mechanisms for data transmission should be as functional, clear, limited, and simple as possible, and the clinical center staff can assist in achieving these objectives.

17.2 TESTING AND TRAINING

Testing and revising the forms and procedures before initiating the trial will generate ultimate forms and procedures compatible with the needs of both the protocol and the investigator. Moreover, special problems at individual clinical centers may be uncovered by pretesting and can be resolved before starting the trial. The number and complexity of forms and procedures should be minimized to meet the essential requirements of the protocol. Morale and performance will benefit from procedures and forms which are workable and satisfy the scientific needs of the trial but are not a burden to the participants.

Another mechanism for stimulation of morale and motivation at the clinical centers is the periodic conduct of training sessions for both professional and nonprofessional personnel. The coordinating center of the multicenter trial should utilize expert consultation for this purpose when necessary. Clinical center secretaries or coordinators who make appointments and complete forms, laboratory personnel who handle and analyze samples, and technicians who conduct clinical procedures almost always find training seminars helpful. At these meetings, the coordinating center can suggest models for the organization and operation of clinical centers, provide techniques for the recruitment of patients, and review aspects of study procedures requiring attention. Furthermore, especially if the sessions are held prior to initiating the trial, useful suggestions are often obtained from the participants.

17.3 COMMUNICATIONS

One of the most important aspects of a multicenter trial is communication, before and during the trial. Clinical centers can conduct the business of the trial effectively only through sufficient telephone and postal communication with the coordinating center, the biostatistics unit, and the central laboratories. In addition, clinical center personnel should have opportunities to exchange mutual problems and solutions. Furthermore, the participants should be apprised of the current progress of the trial without jeopardizing the blind of the study.

A periodic newsletter prepared at the coordinating center and distributed to clinical center personnel can serve as a booster to morale and motivation. It should inform the participants of the progress of the trial, conclusions of committee meetings, problems and solutions at the coordinating center and clinical centers, the recent relevant medical literature, and personnel activities and changes.

Finally, the coordinating center staff can visit the clinical centers or arrange meetings with center personnel to detect and discuss problems. The solution at one center might be applicable to a problem at another center.

17.4 ANCILLARY STUDIES AND PUBLICATIONS

Coordinating center support of ancillary studies conducted in the participating clinical centers which examine the basic mechanisms of the disease or the treatment can stimulate some participants to a high level of motivation. This can be a double-edged sword, however, because of the potential cost, distraction from the main study, and jeopardy to recruitment and to the blind.

A more direct mechanism for professional involvement of participants is the publication of the trial results. I think it is imperative that the clinical center physicians have the opportunity to coauthor publications of the trial. If a cooperative study is adequately conceived initially, publications can be envisioned in addition to those directly related to the basic aims of the efficacy and safety of the agent. For example, separate manuscripts may evolve from statistical or procedural methodology, validation and quality control, description of the baseline population and data, and the natural course of the disease. Ancillary studies provide another source for publications. At the outset, therefore, individuals can volunteer and be designated to assume primary responsibility for specific publications. This will provide a strong incentive for some of the participants.

The final consideration is the funding of the clinical centers. This must be realistic and adequate in relation to the protocol. Moreover, costs vary geographically and among institutions, so that the individual treatment center budgets should be reviewed and awarded cognizant of local costs.

17.5 DISCUSSION

Ancillary Studies

Juhl
Ancillary studies are very important, especially for the younger members of the team. In the Copenhagen Prednisone Study, the main object was the evaluation of prednisone versus placebo in cirrhosis (Figure 17.1), but during the trial several other studies were performed in the patients, such as prognostic indicators in cirrhosis, the effect of continued drinking in alcoholic cirrhosis, side effects of prednisone, and dilemmas in randomized controlled trials.

The Negative Trial

Blum
Many investigators hesitate to participate in a randomized controlled trial because they fear that the treatment under test will prove to be ineffective, and that the negative result will not be publishable thus

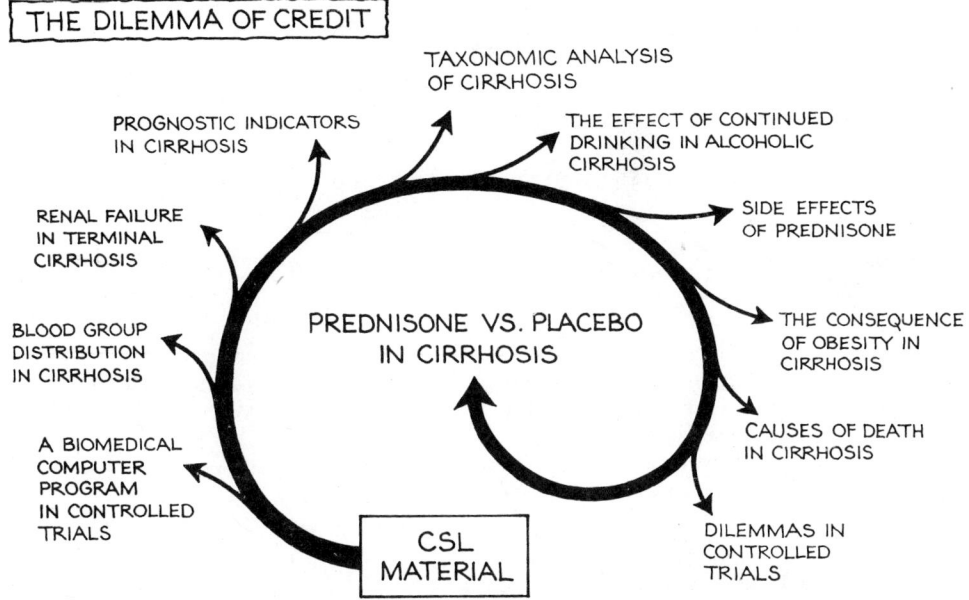

FIGURE 17.1 Ancillary studies performed during the prednisone trial in cirrhosis conducted by the Copenhagen Study Group for Liver Diseases.

neither scientifically nor clinically rewarding. To improve this, editors should be motivated to accept trials showing that the treatment tested is truly ineffective. An editor of a journal once sent me a report of such a trial for review, writing that he actually did not want to publish it because the treatment tested was shown to be ineffective. He was not concerned that it was a well-conducted trial, and I had a hard time convincing him that it was worth publishing.

Riis
It is the editor's responsibility to publish good trials showing no effect of either an established or a new treatment and not to ask for a journal of negative results. Also, the Helsinki Declaration (Appendix B) states that it is an obligation for the clinical experimenter to ensure that his results reach the medical community. It is unethical to subject patients to a randomized controlled trial, and then to distort or suppress the results of negative trials.

Chalmers
Let me put this in statistical terms with apologies to the biostatisticians. The concept of type I error with $\alpha = 0.05$ means that, assuming that there is no difference, in 5% of the trials a chance

difference will appear in a trial when $p \leq 0.05$. In other words, 5 of every 100 studies will reveal a difference which does not in truth exist. Now look at the publications. Which ones get published? Only the positives. Thus, a much higher percentage of the publications may be false positive.

Tygstrup
That is an example of selection bias on the side of the editors.

Lachin
But also on the side of the authors.

Chalmers
Yes, because the author may not write up a negative study.

Juhl
A negative study is as good as a positive one, but unfortunately very few calculate the probability of type II error β or power. A negative study with an assessment of β showing a high level of statistical power should have as high a priority as a postive study with known α. I think it is important to try to evaluate β and power.

Wright
I have never conducted a trial where it has been possible to calculate β or power. I think there are a lot of trials in which it is not possible to calculate β on the basis of the data one has beforehand.

Lachin
I do not see why. Beta does not depend on the data. It depends on the sample size and the minimal relevant difference that one wishes to detect. I see no reason an investigator cannot compute β or power for any experiment as described in Chapter 9.

Tygstrup
Negative trials may be just as important as positive trials if they lead to removal of inefficient and possibly harmful therapies.

Ingelfinger
Well, in my opinion it depends on the nature of the negative results and whether the hypothesis is well founded. If a trial can clear up a misapprehension, I think there is no question that such a result would be publishable, for example, that digitals does does not really help the failing heart. But if somebody administers prostaglandin to see if it dissolves gallstones, and the result is negative, the results will likely not be publishable.

Funding

Blum
Concerning finances, I feel that governments, research councils, and other authorities responsible for economic support of medical research

should be convinced that randomized clinical trials are essential. Otherwise finances will come only from drug companies, and only when they might later make a profit. Drug companies have recognized that randomized controlled trials may be useful, but sometimes they do not like to see published a trial showing a drug to be ineffective. They may sponsor the trial, and if it turns out that the treatment is effective, it may be published, but if it is not effective they may claim that they own the results and they vanish in a drawer.

Lachin
There is an alternative: When funds are accepted from a drug company to do a study, there should be a formal contract between the investigator and the company that it is the investigator's right to publish the data as he feels it is best to do.

Blum
That is true, but usually the contract says that the results belong to the drug company.

Riis
I agree that the medical research councils should take over the responsibility, or if the drug industry is the sponsor, it should be persuaded to give the funds to an independent board for disbursement, instead of the individual investigators having direct financial ties with the firm. In that case one is free to publish the data without having to ask the sponsors for approval.

Schoenfield
This certainly is a difficult problem. The drug firms are in the business of making money, and they have other obligations, they have stockholders. Most often, however, these conserations do not conflict with or compromise the public welfare. In fact, they provide appropriate balance and ultimately may benefit the public.

Riis
The drug industry is very interested in conducting good controlled trials on their products. Negative results will prevent them from trying to market drugs which are not reasonably effective. I believe that they are more on the scientific side than a great part of the medical opinion.

Tygstrup
As a matter of fact, I find that neither the drug companies nor the research councils alone should pay. Those really interested in this problem are the hospitals, and they should also provide funds. I think it is simply part of good clinical medicine to do this, in the interest of the hospitals and the patients.

Lachin
The hospitals can hardly afford to keep their heads above water.

Tygstrup
Well, if we did not use as many useless drugs as we do they might afford it.

ADDITIONAL READINGS

Overton, H. H., Perceptions of the coordinating center: As viewed by the clinic coordinator. Controlled Clinical Trials, 1980, 1, 133-136.

Prout, T. E., Perceptions of the coordinating center: As viewed by the principal investigators. Controlled Clinical Trials, 1980, 1, 127-132.

Relman, A. S., Publications and promotions for the clinical investigator. Clin. Pharmacol. Ther., 1979, 25, 673-676.

Remington, R. D., Problems of univeristy-based scientists associated with clinical trials. Clin. Pharmacol. Ther., 1979, 25, 662-665.

Stamler, J., Effective clinical trials investigators and adequate incentives. Clin. Pharmacol. Ther., 1979, 25, 666-670.

18
Randomized Clinical Trials and the Consumers

THOMAS C. CHALMERS
The Mount Sinai Medical Center
Mount Sinai School of Medicine
New York, New York

18.1 INTRODUCTION

This topic might be summarized with the question: Is all this effort worthwhile? Are we going to be able to convince the practicing doctor that clinical trials should change his method of doing things?

There have been two well-controlled trials which have demonstrated with good statistical power (low type II error) that bedrest has no effect on the course of acute viral hepatitis. In 1973-1974 we reviewed two university hospitals and two community hospitals and found that 49% of the doctors in the university hospitals were ordering strict or modified bedrest (Table 18.1). Of doctors in the community hospitals, 67% were doing the same. This is 13 years after the demonstration that bedrest was worthless.

There have now been eight clinical trials on the composition of therapeutic diets in peptic ulcer therapy, all of which were negative. Of 38 charts reviewed (Table 18.2), 26 physicians, 68%, ordered a bland, soft, or liquid diet, nine physicians, 24%, ordered a Sippy diet. Circa 1913, Sippy, a University of Chicago physician, started a fad treating ulcer patients with a 50% milk, 50% cream liquid diet every 2 hrs, an atherogenic diet, now known to be highly contraindicated in middle-

TABLE 18.1 Admission Orders Written for Patients with Acute Viral Hepatitis

	Strict or modified bedrest	Ad lib or no mention of bedrest	Total
Two university hospitals	58 (49%)	60 (51%)	118
Two community hospitals	48 (67%)	24 (33%)	72
Total	106 (56%)	83 (44%)	190

Source: Ref. 1.

aged men. It never was tested in a controlled trial, but once was and still is popular. Now they use a modified Sippy diet; a little bit of bread or crackers is allowed.

This is discouraging, and it has to do with medical education. In the case of the diet there is no drug company selling the doctors on what to do. We found with oral hypoglycemic agents that sales are increasing in spite of the negative studies. One has to deal with

TABLE 18.2 Initial Dietary Orders on 38 Hospitalized Patients with Peptic Ulcer

	University hospital	Community hospital	Total
Bland, soft, or liquid	17	9	26
Sippy	3	6	9
Regular	2	1	3
Total	22	16	38

Source: Ref. 1.

TABLE 18.3 Conclusions and Validity of Clinical Trials of Portacaval Shunting

Type of shunt and adequacy of controls	Degree of enthusiasm			Total
	Great	Moderate	None	
Therapeutic shunts				
Adequate	0	3	1	4
Poor	9	2	1	12
None	39	10	2	51
Prophylactic shunts				
Adequate	0	0	4	4
Poor	3	0	0	3
None	3	1	0	4
Emergency shunts				
Adequate	0	0	0	0
Poor	6	0	0	6
None	8	3	1	12
For ascites				
Adequate	0	0	0	0
Poor	0	1	1	2
None	8	1	0	9
Total for all shunts[a]				
Adequate	0	3	5	8
Poor	18	3	2	23
None	58	15	3	76

[a] $\chi^2 = 28.6$, $p < 0.001$

Source: Updated from Ref. 2. Reprinted with permission from Chalmers, T. C., Randomized controlled clinical trials in diseases of the liver, in progress in Liver Diseases (H. Popper and F. Schaffner, eds.), Grune & Stratton, New York, 1976, p. 451.

advertising by pharmaceutical firms and with the fact that some doctors are still vehement about the safety of the drugs despite the evidence to the contrary.

Let's turn to portacaval shunt surgery. Initial enthusiasm for shunting depends significantly on the quality of the controls employed in the clinical trials (Table 18.3). Among the randomized trials there is no enthusiasm for prophylactic shunts, and only moderate enthusiasm for therapeutic shunts. In review articles and textbooks, however, the enthusiasm depends not so much on the data from clinical trials as it does on how the writer was trained or makes his living (Table 18.4). Internists and gastroenterologists are significantly less enthusiastic than the surgeons.

Another example is the great deal of controversy about whether radiotherapy should be used after radical mastectomy. There have now

TABLE 18.4 Opinions on Portacaval Shunt Surgery

Type of shunt	Degree of enthusiasm		
	Marked	Moderate	None
Nine textbooks and five review articles by surgeons			
Therapeutic	11	3	0
Prophylactic	1	1	4
Emergency	6	2	1
For ascites	0	3	2
Total	18	9	7
Eleven textbooks and two review articles by internists and gastroenterologists			
Therapeutic	3	10	1
Prophylactic	0	0	7
Emergency	3	6	0
For ascites	0	2	2
Total	6	18	10
Total of opinions by discipline[a]			
Surgeons	18	9	7
Internists and gastroenterologists	6	18	10

[a] $\chi^2 = 9.53$, $p < 0.01$.

Source: From Ref. 3.

been five reasonably well done randomized controlled trials, all of which show no benefit. Yet radiotherapists continue to be enthusiastic. In other words, they are ignoring the data and are advocating their own special treatment (Table 18.5).

Now consider the problem of radical mastectomy versus simple mastectomy plus radiotherapy. There are four trials, all of which show that radical mastectomy has nothing to offer, except for one trial which shows that it is better than lumpectomy in patients with axillary metastases, but not those without metastases. In other words, it appears that a radical mastectomy is not necessary for stage 1 and possibly even stage 2 cancer. However, the opinions of surgeons and radiotherapists on classic radical versus less radical operations again follow the lines of training rather than the data (Table 18.6).

Thus we have a responsibility not only to do proper therapeutic trials, but we have also the responsibility to find some way of educating physicians with regard to the analysis and interpretation of data. That is why I think it is more important, if one had to choose one or the other, to teach our students biostatistics and experimental design than it is to teach them biochemistry.

TABLE 18.5 Primary Treatment of Breast Cancer: Review and Textbook Opinions of Efficacy of Radiotherapy after Radical Mastectomy, 1962-1977

Conclusions	Authors			
	Surgeons	Radio therapists	Other	Total
For	8	24	2	34
Against	15	3	3	21
Equivocal	5	4	6	15
Total	28	31	11	70

TABLE 18.6 Primary Treatment of Breast Cancer: Review and Textbook Opinions on Classic Radical versus Less Radical Operations Plus Radiotherapy

Conclusions favoring	Authors			Total
	Surgeons	Radio therapists	Others	
Radical	19	5	2	26
Modified radical	5	2	1	8
Extended simple	2	2	0	4
Simple	7	6	2	15
Local excision	1	0	0	1
Equivocal	2	0	2	4
Total	36	15	7	58

18.2 DISCUSSION

Ingelfinger
Of course I have been hearing Dr. Chalmers say this for so long that I am utterly convinced by what he says, and I have developed some general principles which I am going to submit to you.

If the result of a randomized controlled trial is consistent with current beliefs, then it is readily accepted by physicians. For example, in the United States, where many doctors were treating hypertension with drugs, a large well-controlled Veterans Administration trial (4) showed that, indeed, drugs prolong the life of males with moderate hypertension. There was no problem in doctors accepting this.

On the other hand, when the result of a clinical trial is not consistent with current beliefs but the result is positive, then it takes time for the result to be accepted. Gradually, the trend is to accept the result, although it may take repeated efforts, perhaps over 5 or 10 years.

If the result is negative and this negative result is consistent with beliefs, then that is accepted. For example, the trial with ascorbic acid (5) in the prevention of colds was accepted readily.

But if the result, as we have just seen, is negative, and is inconsistent with what the doctors currently believe, if, for example, antacids were shown by a randomized controlled trial not to be effective, then the trial's conclusions would not be accepted by the physicians. Therefore, you have heard the law of Laplace and Lasagna, and here is the law of LaIngelfinger: a clinical trial with a negative result, inconsistent with current beliefs, will be ignored.

Riis
This is very important to understand, since this may be the sad reality that we have to face for the coming years. I think it is a problem of which direction this information takes. At present the clinical trial is considered to be a sort of intellectual play, even if it is taken seriously by the small group of doctors interested in this method. The picture will change, I think, when we start educating medical students and young doctors. I can understand the surgeons or the internists who never knew of this method. They receive a message in a language that they do not understand.

Ingelfinger
The problem is education concerning not only the financial interests of the pharmaceutical firms which Dr. Chalmers alluded to, but the ego satisfaction of the doctors. I think many doctors are not purely mercenary, but it is a very stong human tendency to believe in the method that we do, or think we do, best. This is my skill, and if you deny my skill you are denying the value of what I have been striving for. Now, if I am very objective I can balance this bias against the data and accept the data of others, but this is a terrible human obstacle that has to be overcome.

Riis
That is true, but there are different phases in one's professional life. The ethologist Konrad Lorenz's ducklings loved his boots if they were the first thing they saw after leaving their eggs. I think it is extremely important that medical students, for instance, don't crack the shell and love just one pair of boots. They should see several.

REFERENCES

1. Chalmers, T. C., The impact of controlled trials on the practice of medicine. Mount Sinai J. Med., 1974, 41, 756.

2. Chalmers, T. C., Randomized controlled clinical trials in diseases of the liver, in Progress in Liver Diseases, Volume V, (H. Popper and F. Schaffner, eds.), Grune and Stratton, New York, 1976, pp. 450-455.

3. Chalmers, T. C., Randomized clinical trials in surgery, in Controversy in Surgery, (R. L. Varco and J. P. Delaney, eds.), W. B. Saunders, Philadelphia, Pa., 1976, pp. 3-11.

4. Veterans Administration Cooperative Study Group on Antihypertensive Agents, Effects of treatment on morbidity in hypertension: Results in patients with diastolic blood pressures averaging 115 through 119 mmHg. J. Amer. Med. Ass., 1967, 202, 1028-1034.

5. Karlowski, T. R., Chalmers, T. C., Frankel, L. D., Kapikian, A. Z., Lewis, T. L. and Lynch, J. M., Ascorbic acid for the common cold: A prophylactic and therapeutic trial. J. Amer. Med. Ass., 1975, 231, 1038-1042.

19
Randomized Clinical Trials and the Patients

POVL RIIS
Herlev Hospital
University of Copenhagen
Herlev, Denmark

19.1 ETHICAL CONSIDERATIONS

The ethics of the clinical trial affect patients, society, and scientists. The patients participating in a randomized clinical trial are especially affected by the potential ethical problems, but other patients have a potential ethical interest in a clinical trial because it offers the possibility of improved treatment of their disease. Society is interested in the ethical problems of clinical trials in order to protect the rights of its citizens on one side, and on the other to facilitate important scientific clinical activity. Scientists are involved in ethical aspects, because they are as ethically concerned as other citizens, and because they are at the center of any scientific-ethical debate.

If citizens are asked directly, "Do you want scientific activity with human subjects?" the answer will probably be, "Yes, we expect medical science to advance." But if the individual patient or citizen is asked to participate, he may answer, "Yes, but is not my neighbor better suited for such activity?"

For physicians, the crucial question may be whether it is less ethical to do a randomized trial than to prescribe treatments of doubtful or unproven value. This point of view is particularly stressed, because physicians performing clinical trials sometimes think they have to defend themselves all the time. But think of all the stomachs that have been removed, all the mucosal abrasions of the uterus that have been performed, all the tonsils taken out, without anyone asking, "How can I be certain that this procedure will benefit my patient?" So we ought instead to adopt a more aggressive attitude, stating that we cannot go on relying solely on uncontrolled experience.

I consider a methodologically bad investigation always unethical. On the other hand, a methodologically good investigation is not in itself ethical. How then should the ethical aspects of a clinical trial be evaluated? Initially we should always consider whether the expected benefit of the experiment to society is greater than the expected risk to the participating patients, which is always a difficult evaluation.

Many lay people tell physicians that clinical trials are only acceptable if they are of benefit to the patients directly involved. But how could one know beforehand? If we knew that the new treatment was beneficial, the trial would not be necessary; if we did not know for sure, then we could not perform the trial since we could not show beforehand that it would be beneficial. Take, for instance, the first trials on antibiotic prophylactic treatment of unconscious patients. At first many physicians thought that such trials were unethical because they expected that the control group receiving no treatment would be the losers. On the contrary it turned out that this group actually became the winners. There are many other examples showing that what was thought unethical proved to be the right thing to do when the results ultimately appeared. This situation is not uncommon, especially when the difference between treatments is relatively small, and small differences are what we are usually dealing with in clinical trials today.

19.2 THE HELSINKI DECLARATION

How should we decide whether a randomized trial is ethical? Guidance in such matters consists of two elements, one's own personal attitude or personal norms, and the more formal set of rules set down by society (often unwritten). In an effort to develop a general guideline, the World Medical Association in 1963 issued the Helsinki Declaration I, which was adopted in many countries. In the Nordic countries, we in the early 1970s created a working group to revise the declaration, and the revised edition, the Helsinki Declaration II, was adopted by the World Medical Association. (See Appendix B.)

The principles behind Helsinki Declaration II were similar to those found in Helsinki Declaration I; but besides the growing sense of civil rights, the revision was influenced by the women's liberation movement, the youth movement, the ecological movement, and the growing interest in protecting laboratory animals and the world's wildlife. In the following the main principles of the declaration will be commented on.

The introduction to the declaration cites the International Code of Medical Ethics and the Declaration of Geneva, stating that "the health of my patient will be my first consideration." It is stated that the purpose of biomedical research is not only to improve diagnostic, therapeutic, and prophylactic procedures, but also to promote the understanding of disease mechanisms, in other words, the causes of diseases. It is important that the word biomedical has been chosen to characterize the research dealt with. In this way not only clinical research on patients has been included, but also research involving healthy volunteers.

An important statement deals with the fact that every day medical practice involves some kind of hazard, and that biomedical research situations are no exception. A second important statement emphasizes the fact that medical progress is based on research, and further, that such research in part must rest on experimentation involving human subjects. In this way the illusion that medical research can spare human beings and laboratory animals, and, for example, be based on tissue culture studies, is rejected.

Throughout the Helsinki Declaration II an important distinction can be made between medical research with a diagnostic or therapeutic aim, and that which is without direct value to the research subjects. In the basic principles of the declaration, however, it is clearly stated that no human subject should be involved in experiments before adequately performed laboratory and animal experimentations have taken place. It is also demanded that biomedical research projects be planned and carried through according to generally accepted scientific principles. By this expression the declaration refers to the international consensus by biomedical journals in high esteem, scientific societies, and so on.

By demanding the existence of an experimental protocol forming the basis of every biomedical experiment, the declaration tries to ensure that no undescribed experiment takes place independent of public and professional control procedures. Undoubtedly, the demand for such a protocol will have an important secondary effect on the scientific standards of medical research. The same is true for the demand that biomedical research be conducted only by scientifically qualified persons. In other words, when young scientists are involved in projects, well-trained scientists must provide the necessary supervision. If patients are involved, even in psychological or sociomedical situations, it is demanded that a medically qualified person share the supervision of the project.

The declaration states further that no human subject can enter a research project unless the importance of the scientific aim is in proportion to the risk to the subject. When assessing the predictable risks, these have to be compared with foreseeable benefits to the subject and to society. If an impending conflict exists between the interests of the subject and of science and society, the interests of the subject must always prevail.

Not only does the declaration point to the precautions necessary to minimize the physical and mental impact of research projects on patients and volunteers, but also the need to respect the privacy of the research subject. This statement has proven to involve large consequences for research based on human data banks, and the application of data linkage.

Editors of medical journals share these ethical responsibilities. If scientific reports include procedures considered nonethical, such manuscripts should not be accepted for publication.

A patient or voluntary research subject has the right to be informed of the aims, research methods, benefits, and hazards of the project, and the discomfort it may entail. It should be stated explicitly that he or she is at liberty to abstain and to withdraw at any time. Central in this doctor-reserach-patient relationship is the so called freely given informed consent. The importance of obtaining such a consent without duress is stressed with a reference to the dependent relationship between patient and doctor. The difficult aspects of this relationship are focused on by the warning that the refusal of a patient to participate in a study should not have any negative influence on the therapeutic relationship. Special rules are also laid down when the research subject is a minor or a mentally incapacitated person.

When dealing with clinical research, i.e., research on patients in direct doctor-patient relationships, the most important rule is that stating that a control group is acceptable provided the control patients are always assured the best proven diagnostic and therapeutic method. The word proven is crucial, because only such methods for which scientific evidence exists are ethically indispensable.

In the first Helsinki declaration it was emphasized that medical research on human beings could only be justified if its value for the patient could be secured. This was an obvious contradiction, because research would be unethical if one knew the result in advance, but on the other hand one cannot think of a real research project without some kind of uncertainty being involved. In version II the wording has been changed. It is now said that medical research is justified by its potential value for the patient.

19.3 IMPACT OF THE DECLARATION

Undoubtedly, many citizens will consider such a declaration important, but the real test of a set of ethical guidelines for research will be their practical application. In which way does the declaration guide society and scientists? Does the declaration offer sufficient security? Does it have legal effects? Or is it just a way scientists create a sort of humanistic mask for their unchanged use of humans as research subjects?

The declaration does not have legal effects, at least not directly. In many countries, however, the appearance of an international declaration, published and commented on by the scientific societies and the national medical associations, can be said to create a strong prophylatic effect and to possess indirect influence on legal decisions in court.

The appearance of a set of guidelines has not only served a regulatory function but has also had a protective effect on scientists through guiding one in analyzing and evaluating the ethical aspects of a research project. It is not easy to determine, however, whether the guidelines have offered sufficient security to both scientist and subject until further practical experience has been gathered.

One might risk criticism that the recommendations act as scientists' lip service to society, but especially one aspect of the Helsinki Declaration II seems to be an effective measure against such diversionary maneuvers. The point is mentioned in Section I.2 demanding that the research protocol "should be transmitted to a specially appointed independent committee for consideration, comment and guidance." In the Nordic countries the word independent is interpreted to mean that lay people are necessary as members to secure independence. The lay members represent society, especially when evaluating the risks and other ethical aspects of biomedical research on humans.

An important aspect of such scientific ethical recommendations is their influence on the dialogue between scientists and society. In Denmark this dialogue has been rather vivid through recent years. The public opinion is very alert to ethical aspects of research. Undoubtedly, the initiatives taken by the researchers themselves have had a positive influence on the public's understanding of the necessity for research, even with humans as research subjects. When scientists have not fulfilled the demand for public information on these aspects, it is our experience that the media (newspapers, radio, television) fill the gap, sometimes in a positive way, but sometimes in a way not promoting the mutual understanding of citizens' and scientists' viewpoints.

19.4 DISCUSSION

Ethical Considerations

Blum
Is a randomized clinical trial research or an experiment?

Riis
This is a question of semantics. The randomized clinical trial is using scientific principles, and you could call it a clinical experiment, a trial; some call it an investigation.

Blum
Actually for me it is not a question of semantics, it is something very important. We cannot on the one hand teach students to accept the clinical trial as the new way of thinking and the new way of treating patients, and on the other hand apply to it the moral rules which govern all types of experiments. I do not think that a controlled clinical trial is just an experiment. It is a medical act the same as the uncontrolled treatment of a patient, and therefore this declaration has many practical consequences for any course of treatment, for example, in obtaining consent and in many other terms.

Chalmers
The Helsinki declaration is largely referring to medical research. It fails to move in the direction of correcting great inequities by not recognizing that all medical practice is research. Whenever a physician uses a new drug, he is doing an experiment, and one could say that the same principles apply just as much to the practice of medicine as they do to research.

Blum
And not only a new drug, any drug, any treatment.

Chalmers
The thing that worries so many of us, however, is that with more and more rules and regulations about research we may be making it harder to do research. Is it much easier to give a peroral antidiabetic to a

diabetic and take a chance of killing him, than it is to do an experiment to find out whether the antidiabetics might kill him. Based on prior clinical trials, I think it is unethical to do the experiment, but still you could go ahead and give the drug and there is no ethical problem involved.

Tygstrup
In paragraph 5 in the basic principles it was said that the interest of the subject should always prevail over the interest of science and society, but this may be difficult to evaluate. There are situations in which the interests of science and society are so strong that this principle may have to be interpreted carefully.

Chalmers
If this paragraph is strictly interpreted you can never do a clinical trial after the first few patients have been studied, because as I cited previously in Chapter 16, the odds are no longer strictly 50/50 that the next patient will receive the better therapy.

Riis
You can say you have treated three patients and it is your impression that the evidence is still inconclusive. It might be wrong and I don't think the principles are violated in this way.

Chalmers
They are if you make it apply to all medical practice and not just to research.

Riis
We haven't tried to deal with all medical practice. This is a question of national laws and basic medical ethics.

Schoenfield
I have seen it recommended that any physician running a trial should himself take the drug before any patient does, or should undergo any procedure that he is going to give to the patients. This should not necessarily be so. There is some potential benefit and some potential risk to the patient but the ratio would be different in a volunteer or the physician conducting the research where the potential benefit is zero, and the potential risk is present.

Informed Consent

Tygstrup
The informed consent is a very serious problem because it not only introduces a selection bias in patients who enter trials, but also in doctors who participate in trials. The doctor who has read the preliminary reports of a drug and thinks it is a good drug for his patient can use it without asking for informed consent. But the true agnostic has to obtain informed consent when he realizes that he does not know

whether it is better or not, and this introduces a foreign element in the doctor-patient relationship. The agnostic doctor then faces a greater dilemma than the doctor who believes the drug is good in spite of incomplete evidence. Who protects the patient against this type of physician? A more honest solution would be to require informed consent of the patient to any treatment we use, proven or not.

Wright
In England there is now a declaration from the Department of Health, based on a report from the Royal College of Physicians, that any procedure other than a minor procedure, which is regarded as anything more than a venosection, requires the informed consent of the patient in the presence of a witness.

Riis
The original declaration had a discriminatory principle based on benefit. Potential benefit refers to patients. There is no benefit to volunteers, whether they are healthy subjects or actual patients. The patient with a chronic liver disease having a very ingenious cannulation to measure some metabolic pattern in the hepatic veins is running a risk but has no potential benefit. In one of the neighbor hospitals one of my contemporaries said, "We always bring a patient in for an experimental procedure without informed consent because we tell them they are going to have an examination." This is hypocritical, because it is not an examination in the sense a patient understands as being necessary for treatment. It is purely an experimental situation and it should be treated as such.

Blum
In an experiment on informed consent (1), 44 volunteers were asked to swallow a drug; it was aspirin. One group of 22 volunteers was given a 190 word explanation that they were taking aspirin; their comprehension score was 66%, and 13% refused. Another group of 22 was given an 898 word explanation; their comprehension score was 34%, and 45% refused. I think in today's medicine far less than 50% of the medications used are shown to be effective by controlled trials or otherwise. Therefore, more than 50% of our treatments fall under what is called clinical research and therefore informed consent should be obtained. Every patient therefore should actually go to medical school before becoming a patient. The entire burden of uncertainty is put upon the patient, and he suffers more from being forced to give one consent after another than from his own illness.

Riis
The procedure for informing the patient should not be too long or too elaborate. Our experience is that written information should be given together with an oral explanation. If you tell patients something verbally, they are so eager to listen to the message that a blocking effect could occur. Later during the trial they may need to refer to the information that the written document can provide.

Ingelfinger
What do you tell the patients? Is it essential to tell the patient that he or she will be randomized, and how do you explain this to them.

Riis
I simply say that we do not know which of these two treatments is the best, and it is difficult to differentiate them because both the patient and I might be influenced by what we believe, thus we wish to do the trial in a blind way. Neither the patient nor I know which of the two preparations he will receive. Most patients will accept this statement. I do not say, "You may not have the real drug but just an inert lump of chalk." If they ask what the comparison treatment is, however, I tell them.

Chalmers
But how about the method by which you make the decision which treatment they are to receive? Do you explain randomization?

Riis
Yes, we say we do it by chance.

Chalmers
In the United States we are beginning to appreciate that it is not the physicians that determine medical policy. It is the lawyers, and the lawyers have not yet entered into the research field because they are too busy making a living with the ordinary practice of medicine. When they do, there will be chaos, because the legal definition of what is best for the patient is not the scientific one, the legal one is what is done by the average doctor in the community. Therefore, we have to change our laws in some way to get the courts to recognize that this is not the way progress can be made. I have enough confidence in the law that I feel that legislatively we will some day arrive at this, but there may be chaos before then.

Tygstrup
I think there is a real discrepancy between the interest of science and the interests of the individual in a doctor-patient relationship, and we have to find some means of living with this discrepancy. We must accept the fact that the information we can give patients will never prove to be completely true and exhaustive. I feel in general that we should aim to integrate the clinical trial and similar aspects of scientific medicine into medical practice.

REFERENCE

1. Epstein, L. C., and Lasagna, L., Obtaining informed consent. Arch. Int. Med., 1969, 123, 682-688.

ADDITIONAL READINGS

Beauchamp, T., and Childress, J. F, (eds.), Principles of Biomedical Ethics, Oxford University Press, New York, 1979.

Bok, S.. The ethics of giving placebos. Scientific American, 1974, 231, 17-23.

Burkhardt, R., and Kienle, G., Controlled clinical trials and medical ethics. Lancet, 1978, 2, 1356-1359.

Chalmers, T., Ethical aspects of clinical trials. Amer. J. Ophthalmol., 1975, 79, 753-758.

Grundner, T. M., On the readability of surgical consent forms. N. Engl. J. Med., 1980, 302, 900-902.

Lachin, J., Informed consent in clinical investigations. Biometrics, 1977, 33, 761-762.

Lebacqz, K., Controlled clinical trials: Some ethical issues. Controlled Clinical Trials, 1980, 1, 29-36.

Levine, R. J., and Lebacqz, K., Some ethical considerations in clinical trials. Clin. Pharmacol. Ther., 1979, 25, 728-742.

Shaw, L. W., and Chalmers, T. C., Ethics in cooperative clinical trials. Ann. N.Y. Acad. Sci., 1970, 169, 487-495.

Tukey, J.W. Some thoughts on clinical trials, especially problems of multiplicity. Science, 1977, 198, 679-684.

20
Randomized Clinical Trials and the Public

FRANZ J. INGELFINGER †
The New England Journal of Medicine
Boston, Massachusetts

20.1 INTRODUCTION

This discussion has two considerations: the evaluation of the acceptability of the clinical trial to the medical community on the one hand, and on the other to the public. The dangers to a favorable medical opinion toward the clinical trial are the intrinsic defects about which a great deal has already been said. An additional obstacle we have to overcome is the hostile environment, the problem of public acceptance.

It seems to me that the randomized controlled trial tends to be <u>enormous</u>. The design is <u>elaborate</u>, the price is <u>expensive</u>, and its implementation is <u>exhausting</u>. We have also heard that a clinical trial might be <u>endless</u> because we have to follow the patients forever, and we also heard there were <u>ethical</u> problems. So clinical trials have six e's as obstacles.

Now, what about the results? The results are limited in applicability. A clinical trial must focus on at least one major question, or possibly a few, but we cannot be too diffuse in the questions we ask.

---

† Dr. Ingelfinger is deceased.

Furthermore, the results may apply only to the population that was studied. If we did not include diabetics, we cannot necessarily use that treatment in diabetics. The results may therefore be, alas, inconclusive for many sections of the population. So the demand is: Do another trial! But how often can we say "do another trial" in such a difficult, complicated situation?

And finally, results tend to be ignored, especially under certain conditions. As a result, we must have bigger and better randomized clinical trials, and the whole project must be pursued over and over again.

Now, what about the environment? We have the problem that the investigator wants <u>subjects</u>, but the public wants to be <u>patients</u>. How can we make patients want to be subjects? The trend throughout the world is that investigations of captive populations, whom we can coerce because they are prisoners, medical students, or the poor, are increasingly considered unethical. The investigator likes to have patients whom I like to define as <u>administratively available</u>. Patients have to be persuaded now to be subjects, but patients are better subjects if they are administratively available. This means that if a patient has a record in some office, for example, if he is being followed because the government is providing or is paying for his care, then that patient's records are more available, and his whereabouts can be followed. I consider that patient as administratively available as opposed to a person who is taking care of his health by independent means.

In Denmark and in the United Kingdom most people are administratively available through national health service plans. Payment is by the government; they keep records of what is being done. In the United States, however, it is the poorer classes who have been administratively available. Possibly in the future most people in the United States may become administratively available, provided we adopt a national health insurance plan, and provided one can still use patient records within the limitations of the Privacy Act which protects the confidentiality of such records.

But who are most people? Most people are voters. Most people are the public. Therefore it seems to me that in the long run it has to be a matter of the whole public being committed to the principle of clinical trials with randomization and all that it implies. If the voters are so impressed, they will then influence their government. The public has to be persuaded to permit randomized clinical trials; they have to be persuaded to fund randomized clinical trials. This is a crucial point in view of the previous discussion on the problems one has when a study is funded by drug companies. We were told that if drug companies give money to support trials, they may make restrictions on the trials.

The government and the people on the whole have to be persuaded to support clinical trials. And of course they also have to be persuaded to participate, because without subjects there will not be any clinical trials. This may vary from nation to nation, but in the United States it will not make much difference whether Dr. Chalmers or Dr. Schoenfield get up and say we must have clinical trials. They have to persuade influential politicians. Otherwise, politicians will get interested contrarily and argue against the clinical trial. Remember that most of the politicians in the U.S. Congress are lawyers; somehow the medical profession has to impress them with its own ideas. In the United States (and I suspect in other countries) if we can get an athlete or an actress to embrace a clinical trial, then we can sell it to the public. But it is much more difficult to sell it to the Congress.

Unless we can prevent clinical trials from being too monstrous, from being a dinosaur, and unless we can keep the patients or subjects abundantly available, the inevitable result, I fear, is that the clinical trial as we now know it will go the way of the dinosaur; it will become extinct.

20.2 DISCUSSION

Wright

To persuade the public is largely a question of education. I think there are two ways to do this. The first is through the regulatory agencies such as the Drug Safety Committee in the United Kingdom and the FDA in the United States, and the second is through local ethical committees. It is very important to involve lay people in local ethical committees and to get them to understand the principles of the clinical trial and the need to assess any new form of therapy by means of a clinical trial.

Ingelfinger

But FDA decisions do not particularly influence public opinion. It may influence the doctors, but some of the legislators often want to oppose the FDA for one reason or another. On the other hand, many of the lay participants in the United States are lawyers and clergymen, but the lawyers are professors in law schools, and the clergymen are intellectuals, quite liberal groups. Frequently, conservative, reactionary elements, which can include doctors, are not included on the review bodies.

The ideal would be to have two or three legislators or public figures who in a group with doctors could work out a solution to these problems, both financial and ethical. They might then understand that a randomized trial is under some circumstances the most ethical. But unless they participate in long conversations, I think it would be very diffcult. A clinical trial is a difficult, serious undertaking, and if it seems serious to us, how much more serious will it seem to the public!

Lachin

I am also very concerned about the future of randomized clinical trials, especially in the United States. The National Cooperative Gallstone Study cost over $10 million and it will not answer all the questions about the treatment of gallstones. The Coronary Drug Project has cost over $35 million. This and most other large clinical trials are supported entirely by government funds. The late Professor Jerome Cornfield, who had worked in clinical trials for over 20 years, once said that it was only recently that he had been involved with a clinical trial in which the agent was shown to be safe and effective. The other clinical trials in which he was involved had primarily shown the agent to be either ineffective or harmful. Why do we have to do clinical trials at such great public expense to reach these types of objectives?

Schoenfield

Those are easy questions to answer. One does not go into a clinical trial only to prove that something is effective; one goes into a clinical trial to learn whether it is effective and safe. A successful clinical trial evaluates that question.

Lachin

Could not the expense and the size of such trials be somewhat less had we done other research, perhaps more bioavailability studies and more animal studies? Could not the need for some publicly funded clinical trials, such as those which showed established drug therapies to be ineffective or harmful, be avoided by more extensive testing by the industry prior to and after marketing?

Chalmers

Americans spend $100 to $150 million a year on oral hypoglycemic agents; I suspect throughout the world there must be another $50 to $100 million spent on them. The study which showed that they were toxic, the UGDP, cost $8 million to perform. Several other studies could have been done for another $8, $16, or $24 million, and they would have been paid for by a fifth of the annual cost of the pills which people consume.

The studies are very cheap, just peanuts. If you count costs where patients come back to see their doctor because they have had hyperglycemia and because they are on the agent, whereas they would not if they had been treated properly, that is another $200 million. The cost of overtreatment of asymptomatic diabetics is infinitely greater than the cost of any number of studies which would have shown us exactly how, when, and where to use these drugs.

Ingelfinger

But the study has not influenced the doctors' use of oral antidiabetic agents, and right now we have both expenses: the study and the use of the drug.

Tygstrup

I entirely agree with Dr. Ingelfinger's presentation, but for me it does not create a great problem. My attitude toward the clinical trial is similar to my attitude toward democracy. It is full of problems, but I see no acceptable alternative.

Part VI
Appendixes

Appendix A
National Institutes of Health Guidelines for Data-Safety Monitoring in Clinical Trials

The NIH Clinical Trials Committee, has adopted, and recommended to the Director, NIH, to the Office for Protection from Research Risks, and to all institutional review boards established pursuant to the HEW Regulations for the Protection of Human Subjects (45 CFR 46), the following statement:

1. Every clinical trial should have provision for data and safety monitoring.
2. The mechanism(s) for data and safety monitoring should be presented to and approved by the institutional review board as an integral part of its review of the project proposal.

    A variety of types of monitoring may be anticipated depending on the nature, size, and complexity of the clinical trial. In many cases, the principal investigator would be expected to perform the monitoring function.
3. Large or multicenter trials, and trials in which the protocol requires blinding of the investigators, should have a data and safety monitoring unit.

The unit should consist of clinicians expert in the disease under investigation, biostatisticians, and scientists from other pertinent disciplines. Physicians engaged in the care of study patients or directly responsible for evaluating clinical status are excluded.

REFERENCE

NIH Guide for Grants and Contracts, 1979, 8 (8), 29.

Appendix B
Declaration of Helsinki, II

Recommendations guiding medical doctors in biomedical research involving human subjects. Adopted by the 18th World Medical Assembly, Helsinki, Finland, 1964, and as revised by the 29th World Medical Assembly, Tokyo, Japan, 1975.

INTRODUCTION

It is the mission of the medical doctor to safeguard the health of the people. His or her knowledge and conscience are dedicated to the fulfillment of this mission.

The Declaration of Geneva of the World Medical Association binds the doctor with the words, "The health of my patient will be my first consideration," and the International Code of Medical Ethics declares that "any act or advice which could weaken physical or mental resistance of a human being may be used only in his interest." The purpose of biomedical research involving human subjects must be to improve diagnostic, therapeutic and prophylatic procedures and the understanding of the etiology and pathogenesis of disease.

In current medical practice most diagnostic, therapeutic or prophylactic procedures involve hazards. This applies a fortiori to biomedical research.

Medical progress is based on research which ultimately must rest in part on experimentation involving human subjects.

In the field of biomedical research a fundamental distinction must be recognized between medical research in which the aim is essentially diagnostic or therapeutic for a patient, and medical research the essential object of which is purely scientific and without direct diagnostic or therapeutic value to the person subjected to the research.

Special caution must be exercised in the conduct of research which may affect the environment, and the welfare of animals used for research must be respected.

Because it is essential that the results of laboratory experiments be applied to human beings to further scientific knowledge and to help suffering humanity, the World Medical Association has prepared the following recommendations as a guide to every doctor in biomedical research involving human subjects. They should be kept under review in the future. It must be stressed that the standards as drafted are only a guide to physicians all over the world. Doctors are not relieved from criminal, civil, and ethical responsibilities under the laws of their own countries.

I. BASIC PRINCIPLES

1. Biomedical research involving human subjects must conform to generally accepted scientific principles and should be based on adequately performed laboratory and animal experimentation and on a thorough knowledge of the scientific literature.
2. The design and performance of each experimental procedure involving human subjects should be clearly formulated in an experimental protocol which should be transmitted to a specially appointed independent committee for consideration, comment, and guidance.

3. Biomedical research involving human subjects should be conducted only by scientifically qualified persons and under the supervision of a clinically competent medical person. The responsibility for the human subject must always rest with a medically qualified person and never rest on the subject of the research, even though the subject has given his or her consent.

4. Biomedical research involving human subjects cannot legitimately be carried out unless the importance of the objective is in proportion to the inherent risk to the subject.

5. Every biomedical research project involving human subjects should be preceded by careful assessment of predictable risks in comparison with foreseeable benefits to the subject or to others. Concern for the interests of the subject must always prevail over the interests of science and society.

6. The right of the research subject to safeguard his or her integrity must always be respected. Every precaution should be taken to respect the privacy of the subject to minimize the impact of the study on the subject's physical and mental integrity and on the personality of the subject.

7. Doctors should abstain from engaging in research projects involving human subjects unless they are satisfied that the hazards involved are believed to be predictable. Doctors should cease any investigation if the hazards are found to outweigh the potential benefits.

8. In publication of the results of his or her research, the doctor is obliged to preserve the accuracy of the results. Reports of experimentation not in accordance with the principles laid down in this declaration should not be accepted for publication.

9. In any research on human beings, each potential subject must be adequately informed of the aims, methods, anticipated benefits, and potential hazards of the study and the discomfort it may entail. He or she should be informed that he or she is at liberty to

abstain from participation in the study and that he or she is free to withdraw his or her consent to participation at any time. The doctor should then obtain the subject's freely given informed consent, preferably in writing.

10. When obtaining informed consent for the research project the doctor should be particularly cautious if the subject is in a dependent relationship to him or her or may consent under duress. In that case the informed consent should be obtained by a doctor who is not engaged in the investigation and who is completely independent of this official relationship.

11. In case of legal incompetence, informed consent should be obtained from the legal quardian in accordance with national legislation. Where physical or mental incapacity makes it impossible to obtain informed consent, or when the subject is a minor, permission from the responsible relative replaces that of the subject in accordance with national legislation.

12. The research protocol should always contain a statement of the ethical considerations involved and should indicate that the principles enunciated in the present declaration are complied with.

II. MEDICAL RESEARCH COMBINED WITH PROFESSIONAL CARE (CLINICAL RESEARCH)

1. In the treatment of the sick person, the doctor must be free to use a new diagnostic and therapeutic measure if in his or her judgment it offers hope of saving life, reestablishing health, or alleviating suffering.

2. The potential benefits, hazards and discomfort of a new method should be weighed against the advantages of the best current diagnostic and therapeutic methods.

3. In any medical study, every patient including those of a control group, if any, should be assured of the best proven diagnostic and therapeutic method.

4. The refusal of the patient to participate in a study must never interfere with the doctor-patient relationship.
5. If the doctor considers it essential not to obtain informed consent, the specific reasons for this proposal should be stated in the experimental protocol for transmission to the independent committee (section I, paragraph 2).
6. The doctor can combine medical research with professional care, the objective being the acquisition of new medical knowledge, only to the extent that medical research is justified by its potential diagnostic or therapeutic value for the patient.

III. NONTHERAPEUTIC BIOMEDICAL RESEARCH INVOLVING HUMAN SUBJECTS (NONCLINICAL BIOMEDICAL RESEARCH)

1. In the purely scientific application of medical research carried out on a human being, it is the duty of the doctor to remain the protector of the life and health of that person on whom biomedical research is being carried out.
2. The subjects should be volunteers, either healthy persons or patients for whom the experimental design is not related to the patient's illness.
3. The investigator or the investigating team should discontinue the research if in his/her or their judgment it may, if continued, be harmful to the individual.
4. In research on man, the interest of science and society should never take precedence over considerations related to the well-being of the subject.

Index

Administrative structure (see Organization)
Adverse events (see Clinical management; Exits from study)
Alpha (α) (see Errors in inference: type I; p-value)
Alpha postulate, 135
Ancillary studies, 217, 251-252

Beta (β) (see Errors in inference: type II)
Blinding, 15-16, 36, 85, 106, 112-115, 238-241, 243-244
    double, 36, 85
    and randomization, 106, 112-115, 238-241
    of results, 238-241, 243-244
    single, 36, 85
Bonferroni inequality, 183

Clinically relevant difference, 37, 39-40, 89, 122-132, 135-136
    and sample size and power, 37, 89, 122-132, 135-136

Clinical management, 88, 211, 221-222
Clinical significance (see Clinically relevant difference)
Clinical trials
    clinical fundamentals of, 33-41
    contributions to gastroenterological therapy, 21-30
    definition of, 77
    statistical elements of, 77-102
Compliance, 52, 69-71, 86, 209-210
    trial period, 86
Computerization, 93-94, 225-226
Confounding, 154-155
Controls, 13, 15-19, 36, 40, 80-81, 210
    choice of, 36, 40
    historical, 13
    justifications for, 16-19
    nonrandomized, 13
    placebo, 210
Cox model (see Regression analysis: life table)

Crossover trial (see Experimental design)

Data-safety monitoring, 221, 235-246, 285-286 (see also Statistical analysis: interim; Ethics: of early termination)
Decisions, 3-19, 257-263 (see also Errors in inference; Likelihood)
   diagnostic/therapeutic, 3-19, 257-263
   theory of, 6-8
Declaration of Helsinki, 253, 266-274, 287-291
Design (see Experimental design)
Dropouts (see Exits from study)

Early termination (see Data-safety monitoring)
Editing (of data), 94
Endpoints (see Measurements)
Errors in inference, 37-39, 117-122
   choice of α and β, 38-39
   type I (α), 37-38, 118, 183, 187, 253-254 (see also p-value)
   type II (β), 37-38, 119, 254 (see also Power; Sample size)
Ethics, 18-19, 79, 95, 112-113, 208, 217, 235-236, 238-243, 265-275 (see also Declaration of Helsinki)
   informed consent, 112-113, 208, 269, 272-274, 289-291
   of early termination, 95, 235-236, 238-243
   of randomization, 79, 95, 107, 217, 232, 238-241
Exclusion criteria (see Patient selection)

Exits from study, 16, 36, 67-68, 72-73, 91-92, 96-97, 99-100, 157-158, 169-171, 177-178, 237-238 (see also Compliance: trial period)
   administrative withdrawals, 171
   censoring, 99-100, 170, 177-178
   dropouts, 36, 72-73, 91-92, 96-97, 99-100, 157-158, 237-238
   in life table analysis, 169-170, 177-178
   withdrawals, 16, 36, 72-73
Experimental design, 35-36, 78-88, 92, 100-101, 199-204, 210-211
   crossover, 35, 199-204
   group comparison, 35
   unbalanced, 92, 100-101

Follow-up schedule, 86-88, 213-215
   common end date, 87
   fixed maximum length, 87
Forms, 92-93, 222-225, 230-231
Funding, 213, 254-256, 279-281

Harkness dilemma, 240
Helsinki (see Declaration of Helsinki)

Informed consent (see Ethics)

Lasagna's law, 80
Life table analysis, 97, 169-181 (see also Log rank test; Mantel-Haenszel analysis; Regression analysis: life table)
   actuarial, 169-173
   product limit, 178-181

Likelihood, likelihood ratio, 132-135, 193-194
Log rank test, 180-181

Mantel-Haenszel analysis, 161-169, 176-181
Masking (see Blinding)
Matching/pairing, 35, 84-85
Measurements, 59-73, 145-153, 156-157, 160-161 (see also Reliability and validity)
  clinical evaluations, 59-73
  clinical scores, 63-65, 71-72
  direct (versus indirect), 62-63
  multiple, 150
  objective (versus subjective), 148-149
  of outcome, 59-61, 156-157
  prognostic, 150, 160-161
  response (versus concomitant), 146-147
  scales of, 145-146, 151-152
Morale, 214-215, 229-230, 249-252
Multicenter clinical trials, 215-218

Objectives, 78-79, 208
Odds ratio, 164-167
Organization, 219-222, 230
Outcomes (see Measurements: of outcome)

Pairing (see Matching/pairing)
Participating investigator selection, 216-217, 249-250
Patient selection, 33-34, 43-57, 79-80, 208-209
  criteria for, 33-34
  exclusion criteria, 79-80, 208-209
  principles of, 43-57

Pilot study, 226-227, 231-233
Placebo (see Controls)
Play-the-winner rule, 244-245
Power, statistical, 37, 119, 254 (see also Errors in inference: type II; Sample size)
Pretest, 226-227, 250 (see also Pilot study; Training)
Procedures manual, 222-223
Protocol, 92-94, 207-212, 219-234
  elements of, 207-212
  execution of, 92-94, 219-234
Publication, 138-139, 217-218, 252-254, 289
Public opinion, 270-271, 277-281
p-value, 37, 118 (see also Errors in inference: type I)

Quality assessment, quality control, 94, 227-229

Randomization, 34, 43-45, 56-57, 81-82, 105-116, 244-245 (see also Blinding; Ethics: of randomization)
  alternatives to, 244-245
  balanced block, 111-112
  checking of, 56-57
  constrained, 114
  how to randomize, 108-111, 113-114
  restricted, 82 (see also Stratification; Matching/pairing)
  selection bias, 111
Regression analysis, 185-191
  adjustment, 189-190
  life table, 190-191
  logistic, 185-188
  stepwise, 187-188
Reliability and validity, 147-148, 229
Repeated tests of significance

(Repeated tests of significance)
(see Statistical analysis: interim)
Risk-benefit, 16-18, 38, 266, 272, 289 (see also Ethics)

Sample size, 37, 88-92, 122-132, 135-138, 213-218
   achievement of, 213-218
   determination of, 89, 124-132, 135-138
   dropouts, effects of, 91-92
   multiple objectives, 90-91, 136-138
   and power, 37, 122-132
   unequal (see Experimental designs; unbalanced)
Selection criteria (see Patient selection; Participating investigator selection)
Side effects (see Clinical management; Exits from study)
Signal-to-noise ratio, 6
Square root rule, 101
Statistical analysis, 37-38, 41, 95-98, 132-133, 139-142, 150-153, 155-197, 234-242 (see also Life table analysis; Mantel-Haenszel analysis; Regression analysis; Stratification: post randomization)
   dropouts in, 96-97
   interim, 41, 95-96, 132-133, 139-141, 191-194 (see also Data-safety monitoring)
   multiple variables, 96, 141-142, 150-151
   nonparametric, 151-153

(Statistical analysis)
   prediction, 98 (see also Regression)
   sequential, 193-194, 239-242 (see also Likelihood)
   of subgroups, 97-98, 181-184
Statistical inference, 117-143 (see also Decisions; Errors in inference)
Stratification, 35, 45, 49-52, 55-56, 65-67, 82-84, 98-99
   prerandomization, prospective, 35, 45, 55-56, 82-83
   postrandomization, retrospective, 35, 49-52, 65-67, 83-84 (see also Mantel-Haenszel analysis)
Subgroups (see Sample size; Statistical analysis)

Therapeutic decisions (see Decisions)
Training, 216-217, 250-251
Trial period (see Compliance)
Type I and II Errors (see Errors in inference)

Unethical practices (see Ethics)

Validity (see Reliability and validity)
Variables (see Measurements)

Withdrawals (see Exits from study)